"It's important that we women support the black men in our lives in being both physically and spiritually healthy. [This book] will help guide women in taking care of their husbands, fathers, sons, brothers, and friends."
—**DONNA RICHARDSON, creator of the Sweating in the Spirit fitness program and wife of radio personality Tom Joyner**

"As a person who lost the love of her life to cancer, I know how important books like [this] can be in opening up the conversation that could save the life of someone you love."
—**BEVERLY JENKINS, bestselling author of *Winds of the Storm***

"When I go out to speak about black men and depression, three-fourths of the people who show up are women. That's because our women care more about our health than we do. [This book] is an invaluable resource for any woman who cares about the physical and emotional health of a man in her life."
—**JOHN HEAD, author of *Standing in the Shadows: Understanding and Overcoming Depression in Black Men***

"Women are typically the caregivers and health care decision-makers within their families. [This book] is an important tool in the women-led public health movement to eliminate gender-based health disparities among black men. The wisdom and authoritative information included in the book on the range of health conditions that disproportionately impact black men will promote better self-care in our community."
—**LORRAINE COLE, PhD, CEO, YWCA USA**

"This book provides the health information and communication skills we need to help the men in our lives to live not only longer, but also healthier lives."
—**M. JOYCELYN ELDERS, MD, former surgeon general of the United States, professor emeritus of pediatrics, the University of Arkansas Medical Sciences**

The

BLACK WOMAN'S GUIDE TO BLACK MEN'S HEALTH

Andrea King Collier and

Willarda V. Edwards, MD

WARNER WELLNESS

NEW YORK BOSTON

Warner Wellness
Hachette Book Group USA
1271 Avenue of the Americas
New York, NY 10020

Visit our Web site at www.HachetteBookGroupUSA.com

Warner Wellness is an imprint of Warner Books, Inc.

Printed in the United States of America

First Edition: February 2007
10 9 8 7 6 5 4 3 2 1

Warner Wellness is a trademark of Time Warner Inc. or an affiliated company. Used under license by Hachette Book Group USA, which is not affiliated with Time Warner Inc.

Library of Congress Cataloging-in-Publication Data
Collier, Andrea King, 1956–
    The Black woman's guide to Black men's health / by Andrea King Collier and Willarda V. Edwards—1st ed.
        p. cm.
    Includes index.
    ISBN-13: 978-0-446-69772-9
    ISBN-10: 0-446-69772-9
    1. African American men—Health and hygiene—Popular works. 2. African American men—Diseases—Popular works. I. Edwards, Willarda V. II. Title.
    RA777.8.C63 2007
    613'.0423408996073—dc22
                            2006027608

Book design and text composition by L&G McRee

To Darnay Collier, my husband since 1982, life partner, and guinea pig. To our children, Christopher and Nicole, and to Darnay's parents, Jeannie and Willie Collier. Most of all, to the late Louis Comer, who was the most amazing of all black men.

ANDREA KING COLLIER

• • •

To my father, Willard Randolph Edwards, who passed away in 2004. This book could have been of help to him . . . if only. And to my two older brothers, Lionel Edward Edwards and Ronald Lee Edwards. I hope you will read this and follow through on the health alerts that this book brings to the forefront.

WILLARDA V. EDWARDS, MD

Acknowledgments

First and foremost, thank you to every single individual and family who generously shared their stories with us for this book. Each story will help some black woman provide health guidance and support to a man she loves. Your stories may even save the life of a black man—and that is powerful. And a special acknowledgment to the black men we all lost too soon. You are the inspiration for this book and every word in it. The world misses you. A million thank-yous to Dr. David Satcher, for his lifelong dedication to the health and wellness of people of color. Also many thanks to Dr. Henrie Treadwell, Dr. Joyce Nottingham, Dr. Kisha Braithwaite, and the entire team at the National Primary Medicine Center at Morehouse School of Medicine.

Special thanks to the W.K. Kellogg Foundation for providing a lens by which one could see the world of health disparities and the world of the uninsured up close and personal. Thanks to Barbara Sabol for her passion for programming such as Community Voices, and Terri Wright for her work in getting kids care through the School-Based Health Initiative.

Thanks to Dr. Jocelyn Elders; Theodies Mitchell from the Centers for Disease Control; Dr. Jane Kelly of the National Diabetes Education Program; Sheila Jack of the National Alzheimer's Association; Dr. Anelle Primm of the American Psychiatry Association; Dr. Sandra Gadson and Dr. Laura Mathew Thompson of the National Medical Association; Vence Bonham of the National Genome Research Institute; Dr. Lorraine Cole; president and CEO of the YWCA USA; Dr. Richard Payne of the Duke Institute for Care at the End of Life; and Rev. Henry Edmonds of the Bryan Alzheimer's Center at Duke.

An amazed thank-you to Debra Fraser-Howze and Philip Hilton of the National Black Leadership Commission on AIDS, Phill Wilson at the Black AIDS Institute, Dr. William and Bathsheba Johnson at the Luck Care Center in Chicago, and Kaye McDuffie of the Lansing Area AIDS Network for the work you do on the ground to fight this crucial fight.

An important thank-you to the Sickle Cell Disease Association of America, for its efforts to continue to raise awareness of sickle cell disease.

Thank-yous go to Tavis Smiley and Tom Joyner for continuing to flash a spotlight on black men and women and their health every chance they get. Thanks, *Essence* magazine, for putting health in our faces every single month; *Real Health* and *Heart and Soul* and every publication that strives to make us smarter and more proactive; and writer John Head for his courage in the work on depression.

Thank you to the Warner Wellness editorial team, Natalie Kaire, Diana Baroni, and Rebecca Isenberg. Thanks to Jenny Bent, at Trident Media Group. And to Kelli Martin, super editor, now at the house the Mouse built, who helped shape the idea for the book in its very baby step stages.

A life of gratitude to an awesome circle of strong black women who dragged one of the authors through the hard times of this project kicking and screaming, including Mona Terrell, Kimberley Curry Bishop, Nina Moore, Deborah Hollis, Diane Lewis, Jacquelynne Borden-Conyers, Roni Rucker Waters, Dr. Ruthie Jimerson, A'lelia Bundles, Robin Stone, Angela Spears Rochester, Rina Risper, Hilary Beard, Sharon Latson and Dr. Gwendolyn London, Dr. Nanette Reynolds, Lisa King, Melba Newsome, Beverly Jenkins, Marilyn Moore, Felicia Wasson, Eva Evans, Rita Canady, Martha Bibbs, Dr. Rovenia Brock, Dr. Margaret Aguwa, Dr. Marcy Street; and three honorary black women, Barb Mastin, Leslie Levine, and goal buddy Jennifer Haupt.

Contents

Foreword

As assistant secretary for health and the United States surgeon general from 1998 to 2002, I had the opportunity to lead in the development of Healthy People 2010, a comprehensive, nationwide health promotion and disease prevention agenda to improve the health of all people in the United States during the first decade of the twenty-first century. The overarching goals for Healthy People 2010 are to increase the quality and years of healthy life and eliminate racial and ethnic health disparities. By working together to address these goals, as exemplified by this book, we can positively impact the health and well-being of African American men.

In America, we have gained more than 30 years in life expectancy in the last century, from 47 years in 1900 to 77.6 years in 2003. There are more than 35 million people over 65 and that number is expected to double by

2030. While life expectancy has increased for men overall, there remains a significant gap between the life spans of African American men and white men. The life expectancy of African American men is 6 years shorter than that of white men, 69.2 years and 75.4 years, respectively. According to the World Health Organization (WHO), there are factors called determinants of health that affect whether people are healthy or not. These include the social and economic environment, the physical environment, individual behavior and genetics, gender, policies and interventions, and access to quality health care.

Men of color, in particular African American men, suffer disproportionate burdens of health that contribute to their having certain chronic and contagious diseases, as well as mental health disorders, and problems related to substance abuse. Among these diseases and conditions are hypertension, diabetes, asthma, cardiovascular disease, tuberculosis, hepatitis C and B, HIV/AIDS, and other sexually transmitted diseases.

These health conditions, both mental and physical, are exacerbated further by an unhealthy lifestyle as exemplified by the many men who are poor, uneducated, and unemployed, and those who find themselves incarcerated. Historically, African American men and other men of color have been incarcerated at rates disproportionate to their representation in the general population, and their incarceration contributes to their decline in overall health. Of course, African American men are also plagued by a disproportionate amount of gun-related homicides and a higher occurrence rate of HIV/AIDS than white men.

We must take seriously the implications of the status of men's health in America, particularly African American and other men of color. In general, men are less likely than women to avail themselves of health services even when they are insured. Often it is the woman in a man's life who encourages, cajoles, badgers, and uses a multitude of tactics to see that her man attends to his health. This culture has taught men that manliness means ignoring and/or enduring pain, and if you feel well, there's no point in seeing a doctor anyway. Men must release these cultural and societal impositions of toughness and machismo. Men have to be convinced of the benefits of attending to their physical, mental, and oral health.

This book explores ways in which women, by being proactive, can positively impact the health of the men in their lives. It is a ready source of answers to questions about men's health issues and includes personal stories of women's experiences in helping to improve the health of their men. Indeed, these put a face on the men and their challenges, as well as on the women who help them work through those challenges.

The bad news is that poor health outcomes, minimal education, unemployment, and incarceration have kept men, particularly African American men, from contributing as productive members of society and heads of their families.

The good news is that people have begun to address the many issues that affect the health outcomes for African American men, and this book is another step in the right direction. While prevention, control, and treatment of illnesses present a monumental challenge, improving the health of men through early detection and appropriate and timely treatment presents a societal challenge that, if addressed, will result in benefits to men, their families, their communities, and to society at large. *The Black Woman's Guide to Black Men's Health* has boldly taken on this challenge. William Ross Wallace, in his poem "The Hand That Rocks the Cradle," writes, "Blessings on the hand of women! . . . For the hand that rocks the cradle is the hand that rules the world." Let us look forward to the improvements that should result from this valuable resource.

DAVID SATCHER, MD, PhD
Interim President, Morehouse School of Medicine
16th United States Surgeon General

The
BLACK WOMAN'S GUIDE TO BLACK MEN'S HEALTH

Introduction

Why would two women want to write a book about black men's health? We are a writer who has written about issues in health care for over twenty-five years, and a practicing internal medicine physician who is the president of the Sickle Cell Disease Association of America, who has served as the chairman of the board and a board member of the National Medical Association for twelve years, and who is the director of the NAACP's Health Advocacy Division; we both know firsthand that black men are not taking care of their health in the ways that they should.

Studies show that black men who have women in their lives are healthier and live longer than men who have few or no connections. We also know that women are the primary decision makers on issues of health and health care in our families. We select the doctors, set up the appointments, do the research, ask the questions, keep up with the records, and remind them of the recommendations, again and again.

We decided to write this book for you, the strong black women, the pillars in their lives. It is written for the women who love their husbands, boyfriends, fathers, brothers, and dear friends and want them to be around and healthy for a long time. We want them to not only be physically healthy, but mentally and spiritually healthy and possess a sense of well-being.

The Black Woman's Guide to Black Men's Health is the first book of its kind, by black women for black women, focusing on the issue of the health of the black men we love. Look at almost any health-related condition. Blacks in general, and more specifically, our black men, have the highest rates of needless, premature death and disease complications of all racial and ethnic groups in the country. The price of these health disparities is enormous. Not only is there an emotional and psychological impact, but a social and societal impact, as well. In many instances, there can be a major economic impact for a family and thus African American culture as a whole, when a black male head of household dies prematurely at the peak of his earning potential.

Even more important, every time a black man dies prematurely of complications from diabetes, stroke, lung cancer, or heart attack, he leaves behind people who love and need him and will never be quite the same without him.

When a black man dies prematurely, his wife or significant other will go without his love and companionship. His sons and daughters will go without his guidance and strength. His grandchildren, both present and future, will never really know him. His mother will mourn his loss in an indescribable way, because a mother is never supposed to outlive her child. His friends will feel a sense of loss because they will never hear his laughter again.

His acquaintances will miss out on all that he has to contribute. His loss will leave a huge hole in the heart of the black community. There are already so many holes from losses due to substance abuse, violence, and incarceration. These are all the types of holes that not only cause great pain, but also weaken the fabric of the black family that is important to growing a healthy community.

This book, *The Black Woman's Guide to Black Men's Health*, is based on a foundation of "what ifs." After looking at the sad state of health of our men and our community, we asked ourselves some key questions. How can black wives, mothers, sisters, lovers, and friends work together to turn this negative into a positive for our families. What if black women of all ages, all over the country, put their minds to helping to make the men in their lives healthier in a deliberate and purposeful way? What if we were armed with the information and tools to begin to do this? What if black women and men were given accurate, consistent, easy-to-follow recommendations that show what we could actually do that would make a difference in our men's health, be it big or small?

What if, instead of just hearing the same old sad statistics on the state of black men's health, we also heard wonderful, inspiring stories of the power of black women in creating a healthier community?

The more we talked about it, the more the "what ifs" snowballed. What if black women became really even more health care savvy, to the point that they could be viewed as a resource to their families, friends, and neighborhoods?

What if black women and black men stopped whispering about obesity, cancer, depression and suicides, and HIV/AIDS and started talking openly and honestly about these health issues to come up with ways to reduce the toll they are taking? What if we understood more about sickle cell disease, and the need for our community to know that it is not gone, and in fact that it is on the rise (70,000 to 80,000 persons have sickle cell now, which is up from 50,000 persons fifteen years ago). What if we made it a priority for every black man and woman to be aware of his or her sickle cell status, in order to see a decline in the number of black babies born with the disease.

What if we started using our power to shape the attitudes of our sons and daughters about health and their right to health and wellness? What if?

And what could happen if black women became even more insistent, vigilant, politically knowledgeable and active around the obstacles that prevent our communities from having equal access to quality, culturally appropriate wellness care? What if more young black girls decided that their voices and their futures lay in being a part of a medical/health care community that will serve black families well? What if we all committed to carry on the legacy of the Dorothy Heights, Rosa Parks, and Fannie Lou Hamers into a grassroots health and wellness movement to make us all work to create a more equal system of care?

What if black women could bundle up all of our Sister Superpowers—our stubbornness, our gentleness, our resourcefulness, our ability to communicate and commiserate, our ability to love and to dream, and our ability to fight an uphill battle—all to save a black man's life, or to get his life back on track? What if we could do that?

Those of you who have a man in your life—a husband, significant other, father, son, brother, uncle, or friend—know that they sometimes prefer to stay in denial about their health. When a black man finally confesses and tells you that he thinks he needs to see a doctor, all the alarms go off. When he finally admits that he doesn't feel well, we know that he has been ill for quite some time.

We won't kid you. The numbers we cite will speak for themselves. Both of us are involved in the advocacy of health on the local, state, and national levels. We know that if the climate of health disparities is going to change, the political climate around poverty, education, housing, race, and ethnicity must change also. If you have no job, no food, and no place to live, it is hard to focus on acid reflux.

Access to quality care is still a huge issue for black men. We know that if we are going to urge you to get your loved ones to the doctor (not just on Tom Joyner's Take a Loved One to the Doctor Day), we all need to work in the trenches to make sure there are places for you and your family to go.

If we, as the authors of this book, are going to encourage you to get a doctor or health care provider and work with him or her as a partner, then we need to be fighting to make sure that there is a diverse group of physicians to draw from, physicians who may look like us, and if they don't look like us, can relate or who understand the cultural melting pot that *is* us. Evidence shows that when there are people in the health care setting with similar race/ethnicity, the element of trust is increased significantly.

The climate of health care is getting more challenging for everyone, especially people of color. It is going to get tougher to get care, even if you have insurance. Many employers around the country are cutting back on coverage as a moneysaving strategy or to maintain a healthy financial bottom line. And it is going to prove more difficult to take time off work to get to a doctor, and to be a caregiver for a loved one who needs your help, because businesses are now doing more work with fewer employees.

If we are going to address the mental health and wellness issues that plague our community, we are all going to have to deal with how hard it is to get these services at all and then address services that are ethnically and culturally appropriate, consistent and effective for the men in our lives. Women who have tried to do it will tell you that it feels like searching for the Holy Grail.

Black women must also start addressing the needs of the huge numbers of our black men going to and coming out of prisons. They are returning home uneducated, drug dependent, unemployable, and in some cases mentally unstable, because they received no mental health treatment while incarcerated. Many return home with the same addictive behaviors and an unaddressed history of violent behavior, and are oftentimes now infected with HIV/AIDS or hepatitis B or C. Sometimes it seems that for every "what if" we come up with, there is a "but" that also must be dealt with.

The "what ifs" can help us as black women fight the battle on many fronts—especially the home front. The steps and information in this book can make a difference in your home, your neighborhood, and your community, and can impact the information represented on your family tree.

HOW TO USE THIS BOOK . . .

You'll find that chapters 1–5 cover the basics that affect every black man's health. We'll talk about finding doctors, opening up dialogues on health, educating ourselves, and building a health team to address the needs of our men. Then, in chapters 6–14, we will address the top health issues that affect black men's lives, including cardiovascular diseases, obesity, cancers, and HIV/AIDS infections.

Along the way, you will read some very important stories of real women and real men and the ways they have had to face both big and small health issues. Some of the people in the book, such as Deborah Roberts and Al Roker, Tom Joyner and Donna Richardson, and best-selling romance writer Beverly Jenkins, lead high-profile lives. Others don't have a spotlight on them. But in the end all their health stories matter, and they will give you an idea of how real people are dealing with real health issues. Maybe they will inspire you to share your stories with others as well.

A book like this is a tremendous first step in growing future generations of healthy families. It only works if it is read, implemented, shared, and lived. Any one step you take in this book, any pearl of wisdom that you glean can have a major impact on the black men in your life. It may even save a life, or at least, it will certainly increase the length and quality of his life. Together, let's agree that we will work to make a difference in the health of our families by supporting the health of our black men. Why? Because we love them and want to see that they live a long and full life.

CHAPTER 1

Getting Started

If we are paying attention, we are usually the first to notice when something, even if it is "a little something" is wrong with the men in our lives. We know when he "favors" one side or the other when he walks, because of hip or back pain. We almost always are the first ones to notice when he gains or loses weight. We know when he's not quite himself. As we mentioned earlier, studies show that men who have women in their lives are healthier and live longer than men who are single and isolated.

Even though we have a long way to go before we get straight As on our approach to our own health, we do seem to be doing slightly better than our men. Even with issues of ability to pay for medical care, or access to places to get care, women seem to be better at interacting with their health care providers. Why?

THE MESSAGES
OUR CULTURE SENDS

There are many reasons why our black men are not taking the lead on their health care. When we think about why this is, we have to look at the way they have been socialized and the messages that we send them.

Margaret Aguwa, DO, and the chairperson of Family and Community Medicine in the Michigan State University College of Osteopathic Medicine, has developed great relationships with her male patients over the years. Dr. Aguwa says, "From all my years of practice, the thing I could detect in men's faces and demeanor is the apprehension. They are apprehensive about being in the doctor's office, about answering questions about their bodies, and about being poked and ordered around. They are even apprehensive about the instructions and recommendations, even simple recommendations like eating healthy and exercise." Dr. Aguwa says she thinks that it is that apprehension that prevents our men from expressing symptoms and concerns associated with their health and well-being, mostly about taking better care of themselves.

Jean Bonhomme, MD, head of the Black Men's Health Network, says that part of the problem is that black men fear being mistreated in the medical system. There are stories of people of color being mistreated, treated with substandard care, or treated as if they didn't exist, so many men avoid health care at all costs. And sadly that choice indeed has a high cost for many of our men who get late diagnosis and treatment of illnesses that could take their lives prematurely.

As a society, we build high expectations of superhero strength of black men. The message that we send our boys and men is that they have to be strong, no matter what. We expect them to push themselves. Our culture tells our men that they aren't really sick until they are doubled over in pain. You will read many stories in this book of men who did not seek out care and treatment until the pain became too much to bear. The pain was what told them that maybe they should get some help.

The other thing we know is that men and women get different messages about the medical system and when they should seek out care. Women are more accustomed to dealing with doctors and getting the needed attention for ourselves and our children than men, who mostly show up for medical attention in a crisis situation.

WHY IS THE MEDICAL EXPERIENCE DIFFERENT FOR WOMEN?

Let's look at a woman's interactions with doctors. When we are born, we are on a level playing field when it comes to our health. These days most black boys and girls are delivered by a medical system of some kind. It could be an obstetrician, it could be a nurse midwife. From there, black boys and girls are probably seen by a pediatrician or a nurse in a clinic, who monitors their growth, keeps them up to date on their immunizations, takes care of their ear infections and rashes, and calms down their anxious parents.

Then around adolescence something happens. Children of all ethnicities start seeing the doctor less.

They've had their immunizations. They don't get earaches. And they tend not to be that sick. Between the tween and teen years (ten to eighteen), most youth, both male and female, are getting physicals only in order to participate in a school activity or are being seen for an injury from sports. So in fact, during those early teen years, a boy may actually be seen by a doctor or nurse practitioner more often than a girl who is not active in sports.

Of course there are exceptions. Both boys and girls who have chronic illnesses, such as juvenile diabetes, or asthma, which is a huge problem among our black boys and girls, may be seen more regularly to manage their conditions.

Many young black women have their next interaction with a doctor once they become sexually active, if they are planning on using prescription birth control methods, or if they think they have developed an infection or a sexually transmitted disease (STD) that has symptoms. For these reasons, they head to the doctor or to a clinic. Then the next big event that brings a woman to her doctor is pregnancy. Well, this is the true fork in the road for males and females when it comes to their health. There is no event like childbirth that requires a male to seek out medical attention. A man doesn't need a doctor to prevent him from becoming a father or to become one.

The American Academy of Family Physicians says that where doctors usually see women in their peak childbearing years, men don't usually come in for a physical unless their jobs require it, or until they hit their forties or fifties, if then. And if the man is coming in for the first time at that age, you can almost bet that it is at the "gentle encouragement" of a woman in his life. Some men say they got taken to the doctor or hospital kicking and screaming, but they went.

Through watching their fathers, grandfathers, uncles, and buddies, black men actually learn to ignore the messages their bodies are telling them. They learn bad habits that can last them a lifetime.

A Harris study of over 4,000 men and women funded by the Commonwealth Fund says that three times as many men as women don't have doctors. And they aren't getting screened for life-threatening illnesses. The study says that men put off going to the doctor because they are not comfortable discussing their health issues. They tend to show up for medical attention when they are in so much pain or discomfort that they can't ignore the symptoms anymore. And at that point, it could be too late.

Ronald Bishop, MD, is a family medicine doctor who talks to black men about their health on a regular basis. "I think that the state of health for black men is due to lack of early education. We need to get them to understand the value of health care," he says.

"They don't understand that what they do in early years will be a reflection of their health when they get old." Dr. Bishop suggests that women keep hammering home the message that almost every disease is either preventable or treatable, if it is caught early. He says this is one of the reasons why it is so important for black men to develop a dialogue with their doctors.

Dr. Bishop recommends an annual physical for all his male patients—at bare minimum, as a part of good health maintenance. He says that the younger they start with this routine maintenance the better. "I like to get them started at age thirty," he says.

By flipping the script on the way our men interact with health care providers, we can help them get the jump on many life-threatening diseases. A man who knows that he has high blood pressure or high cholesterol can make big changes with our help.

That said, the big question is how do we do it? How do we get the men in our lives to break old habits and take better care of themselves? It is risky business. Often the efforts we make to help are viewed by the men in our lives as a desire to have more control over them. It can become a power struggle between couples and among family and friends.

One adult daughter of a father who was neglecting his health says that trying to get him to take care of himself became very tense. "He hadn't been to the doctor in years, not even for a physical." She says it became a painful battle. "One day he just put me in my place and reminded me who the parent was, and who was the child. It hurt my feelings."

You may have even had these conversations within your own family. They can be exhausting for everyone, and can result in him digging in his heels. Being the health support system for black men who would rather avoid everything around their health can be a pretty thankless job. But as Deborah Roberts, a broadcast journalist and wife of *Today* show weatherman Al Roker, says, "I might be viewed as a nag, but I will own that if it keeps him around for me and our children."

We have to keep reminding them that we are doing

this for their health and well-being. Sometimes these conversations will spin out of control. They become about everything else, from unfinished house projects to overdrawn checking accounts. Stay on target and keep these conversations focused.

BE INFORMED . . .

Sandra Gadson, MD, is the president of the National Medical Association (NMA), and a nephrologist. She says that education is key. The NMA works hard to bring health education materials and campaigns to people of color, as do many other organizations and agencies. Make it your mission to use some of the learning tools available like magazine articles, health books, health features on television, research on the Internet, and sessions sponsored by local health agencies to be more informed about health and health care.

Ask any bookstore staff, and they will tell you that black women are buying and reading more books than ever before. But they will also tell you that although we do buy some self-help books, we're not buying a lot of health books. If you want to be a positive source of health information for yourself, your family, and, your friends (and each of us should be) then you have to read about, listen to, and participate in the information gathered around health and health care for the men in your life and for yourself.

We are not suggesting that you become a doctor, or a health care warden. We are suggesting that you gather and share information that will help you navigate the medical waters for your family and your circle of friends. The experts call it health care literacy, but it's just being knowledgeable about how his body works, how your body works, and what is available to keep them working as well as possible, for as long as possible.

If you read magazines, and there is a great story on hypertension, cut it out. Tell people what you read. If Tom Joyner is promoting his Take a Loved One to the Doctor Day, then put your husband, your dad, your play uncle, and everybody who won't go on his own into the car and take them to the doctor. If *Essence* or *Ebony* is doing a feature on how to cook healthy without losing the flavor and enjoyment of food, try the recipes and share the ones that work with your friends, families, and co-workers. If you see an article in the newspaper about cardiopulmonary resuscitation classes in your town, get a few friends together and take the class. You could receive information that would save someone's life someday.

The Internet is a source of wonderful information. Bookmark credible Web sites that offer sound health information. We mention good Web sites all through this book and there is a comprehensive list in the resources section. Think about forwarding fewer singing, dancing duck e-mails and send more important health information on how your friends can make lifestyle changes that can pay off big for their whole family. In a matter of a few clicks you can reach all the men you care about with a reminder to get a colorectal exam. We both keep reading files of health information from various sources and add to them constantly. More important, we share the information with others who need it.

Take the time to find out what is available in your

community. Know where the clinics and hospitals are. Know where the support services are and how to access them. Invite health service agencies in to talk to your church, your college, or your civic organizations. Invite health care providers to talk to the staff at your job, or at your man's job.

Another piece of good advice is to never draw negative comparisons. The worst thing you can say to a man when you are trying to convince him to make a lifestyle change is to make a comparison between him and someone else—especially if it is not a flattering one. Restrain yourself. It almost never does any good and probably causes hard feelings. If his father smoked all his life and died of lung cancer, it probably is not a good idea to get in your man's face and tell him that he's going to end up just like his father. Instead, try another, more positive approach. Tell him what he means to you and the rest of your family. Share with him how his health worries you and your children. Tell him that you simply don't know what you would do without him.

Offer to be of assistance, instead of insisting on taking control. Let's face it, ladies, we sometimes have control issues. There is often a thin line between helping out and taking over. Sometimes we feel that it is just easier to take over, but the goal is to create an environment where he is in control of his health and you are in control of yours.

The best approach seems to be offering to help. If he says he's too busy to make an appointment to see his doctor, then offer to make the appointment for him. If he has trouble keeping up with his schedule, then take a little time to put his appointments on a calendar for him, or post everybody's health care schedule on the refrigerator. And if it takes knowing the calendar as well as or better than he does, to get him there on time, then do it.

In doing the writing and research for the book, we talked to countless women who love and care for busy men. These are women who don't take no for an answer. Some have gone as far as clearing their husband's schedule to make room for important screening and diagnostic tests, follow-up visits, and even surgery, if it is necessary.

Often it is not totally about the schedule. But the schedule can be yet another excuse for not moving forward. By offering to help him carve out time to take care of dental appointments, time at the gym, visits to the eye doctor, or even much needed downtime to reduce his stress, you can really make it happen.

Helping him make changes does not need to be a big pronouncement. Ladies, we all know that some of the best successes happen with the subtle, quiet gestures. If you want to help a man make lifestyle changes that are sustainable over time, maybe it is better to creatively start adding vegetables and fruits to the menu at home. There is no need to say, "Today I'm throwing out all snacks, or I'm never frying chicken again," unless you want to have a real fight on your hands. Instead, if you are the person who cooks the meals and does the grocery shopping, just plan accordingly. Send him off to work or to school with fruit and bottled water. Be creative in how you prepare food. If it tastes good, and is flavorful as well as nutritious, you will probably get a lot less resistance than if it tastes like a blend of rubber, paper, and grout.

Slow and steady is the best approach when dealing with most health issues, especially when you are talking prevention. The worst thing you can do is read this book and get all motivated to do it all—*Today*! The habits we are talking about changing in our black men's lives were developed over a lifetime. When it comes to lifestyle issues, they may have been developed and practiced over many generations. If nobody in his family ever went to the doctor for any reason, you have to provide education and information gradually, in order to get him to see the value in having an ongoing relationship with a doctor.

Instead of taking on everything, pick one thing to target, then chip away at it, a little at a time. It could be persuading him to get a complete physical so that he can have a better idea of his overall health status and things he needs to work on. It might be helping him address what you suspect to be a bout of depression. He may have put on a few pounds that are affecting his health. If he starts to feel that you are trying to "fix him" and all that is wrong with him, we can almost assure that you won't "fix" anything. What you probably will do is put a strain on your relationship.

The goal here is not to take over his health, but to help him to take control of it. Work on getting him to sit down with you to decide what he wants to deal with first. Maybe his sleep apnea is bothering him and keeping him from getting a solid eight hours of sleep. Or he may be suffering from a nagging toothache. If it is something that he has decided that he is ready to consider tackling, you will have more success in helping him. We want you both to think of this as a health partnership.

Putting Health Front and Center

- Work health into the conversation naturally as opportunities present themselves.
- Cut out and print out articles on important aspects of his health and leave them out, or pop them in the mail to men you care about.
- Go to the church or community health fairs together.
- Be positive. Too much doom and gloom will turn *anybody* off.
- Think about how you would want to be approached if someone wanted you to change a habit (even if it is for your own good).
- Pray on it. There will be times when it seems like you are not getting through to the men in your life. Then suddenly, you'll see that something you said, or something you suggested, got through.
- Praise his progress and support him through his setbacks. There is no place for "I told you so" in trying to help a man get healthier.
- Be an example to your children. Show them that health is a priority in your home and in your world.

Be prepared to make a few health changes yourself. As tempting as it may be, you can't start making demands of another person if you are not trying to take care of yourself and improve your own health. If you want him to try to stop smoking, you have to try to stop, too. You can't get him a membership to the gym and expect him to go if you flop down on the couch after a busy day and do nothing physical yourself. And if you are reaching for the ice cream every night, then it's hard to stop him from sneaking in late night snacks.

Want him to get a prostate screening? Make sure you are getting the screenings that you need, such as a Pap smear and a mammogram, cholesterol screening, and blood glucose test. When you schedule his colonoscopy to detect any precancerous polyps or colorectal cancer, you should be scheduling yours, too. Sometimes you have to jump in first. If you take the lead in your own health and see results, then the changes you make may inspire him. If you start eating oatmeal and your bad cholesterol levels drop, then he might give it a try to lower his, too. If you buckle your seat belt before the car moves at all, then eventually he will. As role models for your children, you will both be showing them how to lead a healthy lifestyle.

Make health a part of your regular family conversations at the dinner table. Weight may be a common conversation topic among families, but the role that it has in our health isn't. Many families have seen the pain that unmanaged diabetes has caused for a loved one, but few families are talking about what is their game plan to prevent diabetes. We tell our children that smoking, drinking, and drug abuse are bad things, but you would be surprised how many mothers never get around to explaining why they're bad, from a health perspective.

Women have a lot of power. We shouldn't be afraid to use it to protect and nurture the people we love. Having these conversations is never easy. And then when it's too easy, you never know if you've gotten through. When you actively take on his health, there will be times when you will be so frustrated. But you also need to put yourself in his place. Positive change is hard and is hard won. But it has to start with us if it is going to happen. When the going gets tough, keep on going. In the end, neither you nor he will be sorry.

CHAPTER 2

Financing Health Care

Self-care and commitment to that care are key if we want to build a community of really well and healthy black men and women. But there is no denying that access to care is a huge issue for people of color. Of course, one of the biggest issues of access is health insurance or lack of health insurance and ability to pay. According to data from the Institute of Medicine, blacks are less likely to work at jobs that offer them health care coverage. They are also less likely to take it, if offered, probably because of the premiums and the co-pays for office visits that still must be paid. This chapter will show you how to maximize health care opportunities, despite these obstacles.

IS INSURANCE ESSENTIAL?

People who go without health insurance or health sub-sidies are often sicker than other people by the time they seek health care, probably because they have put off treatment. They get caught in a downward spiral of illness and debt, which can lead to or worsen poverty. Of course, those of us who do have insurance could easily lose it if we get an illness that makes us too sick to work. In fact, according to the United States Census report on health coverage, in 2001, nearly a million people who make over $75,000 a year lost their health insurance. Millions of people of all income levels go without health insurance each year, due to loss of jobs, cutbacks of benefits, changes in marital status, and self-employment.

If the man in your life finds himself without health insurance, it is important to research alternatives for re-ceiving care. It may mean purchasing short-term coverage, or it could mean signing up for a federally or state subsidized limited coverage program that may be available in the area where he lives. But it is important to find some way to stay in the loop of health care. The more men ignore their health, the more problems develop in the long run.

While there is limited access to care in some urban and rural areas, it is important to know what is available in terms of community-based clinics, community mental health centers, mobile care vans, and free and low cost services available at many churches. Some stores are even starting to offer free blood pressure screenings on a pe-riodic basis.

You can find out about these services by reading the

local newspapers, visiting community centers, watching the local news, checking the church bulletins, and making a call to the local health department. Many organizations post updates on community health events on their Web sites.

Of course, the man in your life would rather have the health care choices and options that having insurance affords him, but many of the free and low-cost clinics in your community are providing solid care. Some health care is always better than none. And there are other insurance coverage options, such as working part-time for an organization that offers all its employees, including those who work less than thirty-five hours a week, health benefits. It could be a good bridge while he secures more stable benefits.

MYTHS OF INSURANCE

Most people think that all jobs come with health insurance benefits. But not every working person has health insurance. In fact, eight of every ten people with no health insurance come from working families. Half of them live in low-wage families. Even if a man has insurance, that coverage may still fall short if he faces a long and debilitating illness such as cancer. Mounting medical bills are one of the major reasons that many middle-income families file for bankruptcy.

As many men who have worked in what used to be considered stable industries like steel mills and automobile manufacturing will tell you, health insurance coverage isn't what it used to be. As every industry struggles with cost reductions, one of the first things on the chopping block is health insurance. If he works in one of these industries he has probably been forced to pay a bigger portion of his employer-sponsored insurance and may be getting fewer benefits from his program. Prescription drugs may not be covered anymore. They may now cost several hundred dollars a month if they are not covered by a co-pay. He may have lost his dental coverage. As a retiree, he may be at risk of losing the health benefits he always relied on in the past.

WHAT ARE THE DIFFERENT TYPES OF MEDICAL INSURANCE?

If his employer offers health insurance, part of his benefits for working there may be paid or partially paid health insurance. His employer collects a premium (payment) from him to purchase medical insurance. The money goes into a fund that pays for medical care for employees who are included in the plan. It is a pool of sorts. Everybody may pay the same amount but some are bigger users of the system and cost it more money. The older a man is and the more chronic conditions he has, the more it costs to cover him. Every company is different in what they offer and how much they charge individuals. The basic types of insurance are as follows:

Fee-for-Service Plan

In a fee-for-service plan, such as some offered by Blue Cross/Blue Shield, or Humana, an individual pays a higher premium because he can use any doctor or hospital he chooses. The provider sends the bill for the office visit to the insurance company, who pays part of it after the deductible has been met. The deductible is the amount that you pay out of pocket for your health care expenses before the insurance kicks in. The deductible is set by the employer or the carrier.

Usually the insurance company pays 80 percent of the customary charges. The employee pays 20 percent. As an example, say your deductible as set by your employer is $200 in a calendar year. You will have to pay out of pocket to your doctor $200 before your insurance pays your provider. After you meet the deductible, your provider will pay $80 of your $100 medical bill, and you are responsible for the other $20. There are no co-pays in fee-for-service health insurance coverage. Make sure you understand your health care coverage premiums and deductibles before you sign on. Also be aware that many insurers set a limit on how much you can spend in health care in a calendar year for certain services.

HMOs (Health Maintenance Organizations)

HMOs offer members of the plan a set of medical services, including preventative care, for a set monthly premium and a co-pay. The HMO plans give members a list of doctors from which they must chose a primary care provider. This doctor then becomes the health care gatekeeper for all tests, screenings, and referrals to specialists. He or she manages and coordinates all other care. An HMO covers the costs of physicians and services inside the HMO group. Without a referral from your primary care provider, any costs you incur for treatment out of the HMO network will not be covered. The patient is responsible for paying the cost of services. You will pay a co-pay for each doctor visit and prescription that is covered within that plan. If you require a prescription that is outside of the list of approved medicines, you will have to pay for it out of your own pocket.

Managed Care Plans/PPOs

Preferred Provider Organizations (PPOs), such as Physician's Health Plan, have arrangements with hospitals, doctors, and labs to accept lower fees for services from the insurance company. The biggest difference is that the network of doctors, hospitals, laboratories, and other care providers in a PPO is usually larger than that of an HMO. You can pick any doctor in the PPO network. A participant in a PPO usually pays a lower premium than he pays in a fee-for-service plan. But he also pays a co-pay each time he accesses the system. If he goes to the doctor for a physical, his co-pay will be $10 (depending on the plan) and if he has to fill a prescription, he might pay $5 to $10 for each drug covered under his plan. He will pay 100 percent of the cost of a prescription not covered in his plan. Make sure you study the list of providers and services offered in that particular PPO before making a decision. Just like the HMO, if you require a prescription that is outside of the list of approved medicines, you will have to pay for it out of your own pocket.

ASIDE FROM AN EMPLOYER, HOW ELSE DOES A PERSON GET INSURED?

The majority of people who have health or dental insurance coverage receive it through their jobs or the job of a family member. If a man is self-employed or his company does not offer health insurance, he can buy individual health insurance, which can be extremely expensive. Most times these policies cost more than group insurance policies offered by employers, and cost men with families more than $1,000 a month. Sometimes people can become a part of a professional organization, a union, or a group like AARP, which offers reduced rate insurance to their members.

Another option is county health plans that are subsidized insurance offerings. As an example, in Ingham County, Michigan, the Ingham Health Plan provides limited health care services for men and women who are living without coverage or ability to pay for care. There are many of these popping up around the country. Call your local health department to see if there is a similar program available in your area.

SELECTING A PLAN

If he is employed and is offered health coverage, a male may have some choices to make. Usually when a person is hired into a company that offers health benefits, he or she is asked to choose from their menu of plans. One of his choices could be using an HMO or a PPO. It is important to spend time researching the offerings and comparing them to his needs and his personal situation. If he knows that he has a relationship with a family practice doctor or specialist that he would like to continue seeing, he needs to make sure that the plan he is considering allows him to continue seeing that doctor.

Does he have medications that need to be covered in the plan? If he or his family have specific medicines that must be used, then make sure the plan covers those medications. Some medicines, say, for cholesterol, can cost over $100 per month, if they have to be purchased out of pocket, versus paying a $5 or $10 co-pay.

Does the plan offer hospitalization? Is that hospitalization paid for at 100 percent of costs? Is it paid out at 80 percent of costs? Make sure that you and the man in your life understand the costs involved before a decision is made on coverage.

MEDICAID

Medicaid provides health care coverage to low-income people and disabled persons. It is funded by a combination of state and federal dollars. It is not all that easy for a man to get coverage under Medicaid unless he is blind or disabled, or is receiving supplemental security income assistance. States also cover medically needy individuals who would ordinarily be eligible for Medicaid but their income is higher than the eligibility requirements. For more information about Medicaid eligibility, call your local Social Security office, or go online to www.cms.hhs.gov/medicaid/statemap.asp.

MEDICARE

Medicare is a federal health insurance program available to Americans who are age sixty-five and older. People with certain disabilities qualify for health care coverage under Medicare. Medicare is becoming more complicated to figure out each and every day. And with the changes in prescription drug coverage, many community centers and outreach groups are helping seniors figure out the best options for them.

An individual doesn't automatically receive Medicare. He has to enroll. Social Security personnel suggest that he shouldn't wait until he turns sixty-five to sign up, but do so three months before his sixty-fifth birthday. If for some reason he signs up later than his birthday, it could delay his coverage. If he is Medicare eligible, he needs to go to his local Social Security office, or sign up right online. To enroll go to www.medicare.gov or call the Social Security Administration offices at 1-800-633-4227.

In cities and counties around the country, policy-makers have been wrestling with creative ways to offer health care coverage to the uninsured. Some have created a complex system to make limited preventative and treatment care available to individuals and families who cannot afford to pay for service or for premiums (many do pay a small co-pay for office visits and prescription medicines).

BE AN ADVOCATE/DETECTIVE FOR A MAN WITHOUT INSURANCE

One of the best things the black women in a community can do is to understand the resources available for the uninsured and underinsured individuals and families where they live. Don't be afraid to call the hospitals, local clinics, community centers, religious groups, and social services offices to find out what kind of funds are available to pay for needed medical services. Some clinics and hospitals have programs that offer discounted or free services to the uninsured or underinsured. Check to see what's available in your area. Navigating the health care system is a hard road. If you've ever had to chase a medical bill around, you know this is true.

You may read this and say that this is something that you don't have to worry about for you or the men in your life. We say that you do. You never know. People get laid off, downsized, and fired, or they become too sick to work. Money becomes tight, and people are making tough choices between chemotherapy and keeping the lights on. Men who need their high blood pressure medicine are buying groceries and gas for the car instead.

You may not know all there is about insurance and

care, and which providers accept what, but you definitely need to help create a network where you know who to ask.

ADDITIONAL TYPES OF HEALTH INSURANCE

There are several types of other insurance with varying degrees of coverage. If you are helping a man in your life determine what kind of health insurance is best for him and his family, the information that follows may be helpful.

Disability Insurance

At any given age the odds of a man becoming disabled are much higher than dying. One of every seven workers will suffer a five-year or longer period of disability before age sixty-five, and if he's thirty-five now, his chances of experiencing a three-month or longer disability before reaching age sixty-five are 50 percent. Most of us don't have the financial reserves to tide us over in the event of a disability that prevents us from working, or causes us to deplete resources in medical expenses. The bottom line is that if he's working and needs his income to live, he needs disability insurance.

Usually, if he becomes disabled under this kind of coverage, he will receive between 50 percent and 60 percent of his monthly earned income before taxes. (Unearned or investment income does not qualify because it continues even if you are disabled.) You cannot get more coverage than that because the insurance company does not want to deter you from returning to work.

Social Security Benefits for Disability

Social Security is another option. It does not just provide retirement income when a person retires, but disability income as well. The bad news is that it's very difficult to qualify for Social Security disability benefits. More than 80 percent of the applicants are refused the first time around.

If your loved one would like to get an estimate of what his Social Security disability benefits might be, have him call his local Social Security office or go to www.ssa.gov.

Just as with retirement benefits, your disability income is dependent upon your "covered earnings," or the amount on which you are taxed for Social Security. Social Security disability benefits are great to have if you can qualify, but don't count on them when you evaluate your disability income needs. And even if you do qualify, the benefits probably won't be enough for you and your family to maintain even the most basic standard of living.

Workers' Compensation

Most employers are required to provide workers' compensation coverage. The amount and duration of monthly benefits vary by state. The coverage only pays for a job-related disability, typically lasts for only a few years, and the payments are low. Just as with Social Security disability payments, it's wise to think of workers' compensation as a nice "extra" if you qualify, but don't count on it.

Long-Term Coverage

If the man in your life will need any kind of long-term nursing care, you need to know that good care doesn't come cheap. The yearly cost of a one-year nursing home stay is almost $50,000, and none of this cost is covered by Medicare, Medigap, or private medical insurance. Even home health care, the least expensive alternative for someone who needs regular medical attention, costs an average of more than $1,000 a month—more if you live in an urban area.

Many employers now offer long-term care insurance as an optional employee benefit. Usually the employee, the employee's spouse, and the employee's parents are eligible to buy coverage. You can save money also by choosing a policy with a longer waiting period, lower benefits, or coverage that ends after a certain time frame. However, as with life insurance, the amount of the premiums is not the most important consideration when purchasing long-term care insurance—in fact, it is one of the least important considerations.

Things You Need to Know Before Purchasing a Long-Term Care Policy

- Purchase a policy that is "qualified," because only these policies allow you to take a tax deduction for the premiums, and pay out tax-free benefits.
- Make sure the insurance company cannot cancel your policy if it finds out that you're in poor health. Note that virtually no companies issue policies with guaranteed premiums, because no one can predict future health care costs.
- Find a plan with a waiting period no longer than three months before being able to access health care coverage, and you should only have to meet that requirement once during your lifetime.
- Ask if the policy covers home health care, as well as skilled, intermediate, and custodial nursing home care. These provisions give you an option to stay at home and receive care, as well as to receive all levels of care in a nursing home. That way, if your condition changes, you don't lose any benefits.
- Buy a policy that does not require hospitalization before the coverage for other services begins. A man may simply start needing home health care, and his medical insurance might not pay for this service without a hospital stay, in which case you would have to pay out of pocket for a home health care visit.
- Make sure coverage includes cognitive impairment of any kind as well as Alzheimer's disease. Other triggers should include the inability to perform two out of five or six activities of daily living (ADL)—usually eating,

bathing, dressing, using the toilet, transferring (moving unassisted from a bed to a chair), and continence.

• Find out about the cost of these health care services in your area so that you can choose a policy that adequately covers those costs. Your insurance agent, or a state elder-care agency, should be able to give you this information.

• Make sure your policy benefits will keep up with rising costs of home health and nursing home care. Your agent or state elder-care agency can help.

• If possible, purchase a policy with a benefit period that covers six years or more of a long-term stay. The benefit period should be the same for nursing home care and health care.

• Look for a policy with no pre-existing condition clause.

• Be aware that a traditional long-term care policy is based on reimbursement of eligible expenses—you submit actual expenses and get reimbursed. Other policies are indemnity based—if you qualify for benefits, you receive the daily benefit and pay for your expenses with it. You don't submit bills for approval.

• Make sure you buy insurance from a company that has been selling long-term care insurance for at least five years.

• Ask for a sample copy of the exact contract of the policy you would be purchasing from your company. Here is where you will probably get the answers to most of the questions listed above. Do not depend on what an insurance agent tells you verbally; it's what's in the contract that counts.

DENTAL INSURANCE COVERAGE

Dental insurance works in much the same way that medical insurance works. For a specific monthly rate (premium), you are entitled to certain dental benefits, including regular checkups, cleanings, X-rays, and certain services required to promote general dental health. Some plans will provide broader coverage than others and some will require a greater financial contribution on your part when services are rendered. Some plans may also provide coverage for certain types of oral surgery, dental implants, or orthodontia.

Some plans, however, exclude or discourage necessary dental treatment such as sealants, pre-existing conditions, adult orthodontics, specialist referrals, and other dental needs. Some also exclude treatment by family members. Patients need to be aware of the exclusions and limitations in their dental plan but should not let those factors determine their treatment decisions. Discuss your family's current and future dental needs with your dentist before making a final decision on your dental plan.

THINGS TO DO

Review your man's health insurance coverage with him. Most health insurance providers allow you to make changes once a year or with a change of family status such as marriage, the birth of a child, or divorce. Review the following:

- If he is planning on retiring, make sure he understands the retirement health care benefits he is being offered, especially if he is taking an early retirement.
- If he has been laid off or downsized from his job, immediately review the severance package (if there is one) for the health care coverage. Some companies are severing health coverage effective the moment of the layoff notice. If he negotiates a longer coverage period, he needs to get it in writing and signed by all parties.
- Know what is available in the way of health care coverage alternatives within your city and state.

CHAPTER 3

Finding the Right Doctor

Many men of color do not have a doctor who they rely on and trust. There are many reasons for this, including lack of insurance. Ronald Bishop, MD, a Michigan-based family practice physician, paints a telling example of how this can play out.

"Say you are a man without health insurance, and you get a sore throat. With no insurance the treatment could easily cost $150 between the prescription and the office visit. Then the doctor says, come back in two weeks for follow-up. That will cost him even more money," Dr. Bishop says. "So you can see why men without insurance may not be able to afford that kind of cash output." This is just for a sore throat. Imagine the costs of an injury, the tests to determine if he has had a heart attack, or the treatment for cancer.

No matter what his circumstances are, we must still

push to get him to begin a relationship with a doctor. Without a doctor who is monitoring his health, recommending screenings and tests in an age- and risk factor–appropriate manner, he is more likely to fall between the cracks of good health. Men who do not have a relationship with a physician or health care provider are more likely to have medical conditions that are undiagnosed and untreated. They are also more likely to have the advanced stages of a disease when it is finally diagnosed. Having a good health care provider on his team, and you as his advocate, can greatly improve a man's health in the long run.

Unfortunately, many men of color, especially the uninsured, are seeking out their primary care in the emergency rooms in this country. In many cases, it *is* an emergency by the time that they seek medical care. But in other cases, it is a matter of not being able to get care elsewhere.

There are several reasons for this, including the fact that many black men do not have an ongoing relationship with a doctor, if they have a doctor at all. Also, most medical practitioners will not see patients in their offices without some form of health insurance coverage or ability to pay. In fact, many families report that trying to find providers who will accept Medicaid coverage at all is a challenge. The emergency rooms provide important, lifesaving care for patients every minute of every day. But they should not be used to meet a patient's primary care needs.

While some people go to the emergency room because they think they will get seen faster, the truth is that ER personnel place priority on emergencies, such as accident victims, people who are possibly suffering from heart attacks or stroke, and of course, injuries due to violence such as gunshots and stabbings. It should also be remembered that emergency room care is not a free alternative. If you've ever seen an ER bill, you know that it is more expensive to receive care there than paying out of pocket in a doctor's office, or finding a low-cost or no cost clinic. As we have mentioned before, an alternative for those who do not have a doctor or for those who do not have health coverage is the local health department or community-based care clinic available in your area.

Many times the emergency room is the only place your loved one can be seen if he does not have the ability to pay or is not covered by private health care insurance, or if he has an after hours illness or injury situation. Many black seniors and parents of young children are also using the emergency room as the place where they seek out routine care.

It is more difficult than ever to find a doctor for your family. And if you are looking for the "right doctor" for the man in your life, then it is even more difficult. In many situations, say, if you belong to a Health Maintenance Organization (HMO) or Preferred Provider Organization (PPO), you may just sign with whoever is available and accepting new patients. If he is getting his care at a local health clinic, then he may be limited to the physicians on staff at that particular time.

The optimum is to get your man matched up with the right doctor for his needs. There are a lot of elements that go into selecting a health care provider.

Gender can play a role in those relationships. Right or wrong, not all men are comfortable with sharing the most intimate details of their health with a female physician. A man we talked to about this said that he could never have a prostate or digital rectal exam if it was done by a female physician. If this is how your man feels, just respect his concerns, and don't let his feelings be an obstacle in the way of his seeking care.

Other men have problems with the language barriers, and stop going because they don't understand what the doctor is saying to them.

Even though there is a shortage of doctors in this country, you should still encourage and support your man in finding a doctor he trusts. Choosing a doctor is such a personal decision with many feelings involved. It explains why so many men shy away from office visits for as long as possible. The fear and anxiety of going to the doctor can be so strong that it can even temporarily raise a person's blood pressure above normal levels. Experts call it "white coat hypertension."

If a man goes to his doctor full of anxiety and fear, and then he is not treated with respect, or feels that he is not heard, then of course, he won't want to come back—ever. All the work you may have done to get him to the doctor can be undone by a rude receptionist, or a doctor who refuses to answer his question, avoids shaking his hand, or talks to him in a condescending way. The best way to avoid this is to find a good match early on.

Dr. Bishop says that once a man is comfortable with his doctor, it becomes a lot easier to build a relationship. "It really is in the hands of the doctor to establish a bond with his patients. It's not an easy task. And some doctors are better at it than others."

SHOPPING FOR CARE . . .

Realistically speaking, most men will not "shop" for a doctor themselves. They will go to whoever is available, unless they have one of those gender biases we talked about earlier. Case closed. Of course, if he's lucky, a man has a provider he likes and has had for years. But this is rare in the age of managed care. A provider who knows you and has a relationship with you is the best possible option. If your provider moves, retires, or if you decide for some reason that there is a need for a change, the chances are great that the information gathering, getting referrals, and trying to schedule a new appointment will probably fall on your shoulders, on your man's behalf.

Just as you would have a list of needs and wants when you go shopping for a car, a place to live, or a school for your children, you should probably be armed with a list of things that are important to your man (and you if you will be seeing the same provider) before you shop.

Here are some important things to consider when helping him select his doctor:

• Does he or she accept your insurance coverage? If not, is payment due at time of service? How will you pay for services? Cash or credit card?
• How does the office staff greet patients on the phone and in person? Are you treated with respect and kindness? Are they helping you get referrals when needed?
• Do you feel as though they are making assumptions about you based on your race or ethnicity?

• Do they follow up on test results? How willing are they to take time to explain test results and treatment?
• What screening tests can be done in the office and what tests do they routinely send patients to other facilities to have done? How does this impact the timing of receiving the test results?
• Do they return calls in a reasonable time frame?
• Do they provide you with contact information for after-hours care and emergencies?
• Do they talk about prevention and share information on recommended screenings?
• How close is the office or clinic to where he lives? Is transportation an issue? Is the office wheelchair accessible if that's an issue?
• Do patients wait for minutes or hours in the reception rooms and waiting rooms?
• Do they provide prescription samples along with the prescription?
• Do they write prescriptions for generic options when available and suitable, to help save you money on meds?
• Are there language barriers between your man and the doctor or staff that keep them from communicating with one another?
• Are they in touch with your culture's medical concerns and issues?
• Do they have hospital admitting privileges? Where?

Now that you've developed a list of questions, help the man in your life look before he actually needs the doctor. The worst time to start looking is when he needs to get in right away. You can check local lists of physicians and check with your HMO or PPO to see who is taking new patients. But one of the best ways to find a doctor is to ask your friends and family who they are going to and why they do and don't like the care they receive there. They can give you personal insights into their experiences with the things on your health care shopping list.

Health care providers normally attend to the scheduling needs of their existing patients before they work in new patients. Suggest that your man use an initial visit to get to know the doctor and to let the doctor get acquainted with him. He will be able to tell quite a bit about how comfortable he feels in that first visit.

Just like any relationship, the bond between a doctor and a patient is built over time. Hopefully, the man in your life will feel comfortable with and have confidence in the provider he has selected. But if he doesn't and it is the reason he is not seeking medical attention, he should move on. If his questions are not being answered, or his concerns are not being heard, it may be time for a new health care provider.

You can offer to go with him if he is feeling nervous or unsure about his visit, but it isn't necessary. Some men really want and need to have that private relationship with their doctors. They may want to ask questions they wouldn't ask if you were in the room. If you want to encourage his involvement with his health care provider, you have to listen to what he's saying about how he feels comfortable receiving that care.

WHERE TO FIND A DOCTOR . . .

Sometimes it will feel like finding the right doctor, or if you live in an area that has a shortage of doctors, any doctor at all, is like searching for a needle in a haystack. As we said, if you are enrolled in an HMO or PPO group, you may be limited to choosing a provider within that network who is accepting new patients. But here are some other suggestions:

- Get recommendations from friends, family, or co-workers.
- Check with the National Medical Association's Physician Locator Service at www.nmanet.org or the American Medical Association's Physician Finder Web site at www.ama.org or call them at 312-464-5000.
- Check with your local department of health, especially if they provide clinical services.
- Call the medical teaching institutions within the universities in your area.

SECOND OPINIONS

Willard Walker was an in-charge guy, until he was diagnosed with macular degeneration and a torn retina that needed surgery. But it didn't take long to find out that the surgery hadn't worked.

"My wife, Quintella, and I went for a consultation with the doctor who had been treating me," he says.

"The doctor told us that he had looked at the options and that there was nothing out there to save my eye."

Willard was stunned, but was willing to accept what the doctor had to say. "I figured that there was nothing I could do. After all I had two eyes. If I had to lose one . . ." he says.

But Quintella wasn't ready to accept the diagnosis. She did her homework and in talking to family and friends, she was able to connect Willard with Greer Geiger, MD, a black female eye doctor who was based in Birmingham, Alabama, and had success with the toughest eye cases, like Willard's. They got a second opinion from Dr. Geiger, who felt that she could help them through a delicate eye surgery procedure. And she did. When Willard says, "If it hadn't been for Quintella, I would have definitely lost that eye," Quintella says—with conviction—"He's right."

What should a man do when he receives a life-threatening diagnosis, or a recommendation for treatment of an illness that may call for surgery, or complex treatment like chemotherapy, or as in Willard's case, the loss of an eye?

He should request a referral for a second opinion, if it is not automatically offered by his physician. Why? One of the main reasons is that the practice of medicine changes so quickly. It would be virtually impossible for any one health care provider to have all the answers.

The second opinion is the backup plan. It gives a patient confidence that the treatment plan or the surgery is the right course of action for him. In many cases, a second opinion could mean that a recommended surgery might not be necessary to treat a given disease. The doctor who gives the second opinion may suggest medications instead. And in some cases, this doctor may find that the patient does not have the illness at all.

Second opinions are vital for many reasons. New procedures to treat specific illnesses are being developed at different medical facilities all the time. Another reason is that errors do sometimes occur. Practitioners and lab technicians are human beings. As many as 10 percent to 20 percent of second opinion diagnoses and treatment plans differ significantly from the original.

If the man in your life has not sought out a second opinion, he is not alone. A recent survey of adults showed that more than 30 percent had never sought a second opinion for a medical problem.

Many men opt not to have a second opinion for fear of seeming disloyal to or to be questioning the authority of their doctor. Others forgo a second opinion because they are not aware that many insurers cover this option. But it is important to ask your health insurance provider if a second opinion is an option.

Here are other questions you might want to ask if the man in your life is facing a surgery:

- What is the surgery for, and is it really needed?
- Is there another treatment that would be as effective as surgery?
- What are the risks of this procedure?
- What happens if a decision is made not to have the surgery?
- Will the surgery improve his quality of life?

Don't forget that the second opinion is an important part of the medical records. Make sure that someone is taking notes and adding it to your files at home for future reference.

CHAPTER 4

Prescription Drugs

Americans take more medicine than people in any other part of the world. It seems like there is a prescription drug or over-the-counter medicine for any possible illness or discomfort that you can think of. Between private insurance, government programs, and out-of-pocket expenses, the 2003 spending for prescription medications in the United States was nearly $200 billion. With all those pills it becomes hard to keep up with the spiraling costs of medicine.

Picking a pharmacist who will help your man manage his prescriptions is an important part of building his health care team. If you or the man in your life picked a pharmacist the way that most people do, you probably settled on some place that was convenient. The drug store may be around the corner, which can be an important consideration if transportation is an issue. In the age of superstores that sell lettuce, Viagra, and televisions, you and he may have selected the pharmacy in the store where you purchase your groceries on a weekly or monthly basis.

With the rising costs of medications, and fewer drugs being covered, price is also a factor, especially if the medicines you take are not covered by a uniform co-pay. Although many families and individuals have a co-pay through their private insurer, or through Medicaid or Medicare, shopping for the lowest price can be an issue if you are paying out of pocket.

Let's look at the pharmacist as more than just the person who doles out the pills. Consider him or her as an important member of the health care team. In the age of managed care, doctors come and go. Many men have had the experience of having a new health care provider every time they go to the clinic or medical center.

The pharmacist can be the one consistent link to health care that you have. If you thought that this person and his or her ability to do the job of getting the right prescriptions with no life-threatening errors could save your son's life, or put your father's in jeopardy, would you look at the process of choosing the pharmacist differently?

Given the role that medications are playing in managing our illnesses, the pharmacist is more important than ever before. It's time to understand what the pharmacist does, and maximize what he or she can do to keep the men in your life healthy.

PICK A SPOT AND STICK TO IT . . .

One of the best tips we can share with you is don't pharmacy hop. Pick a pharmacy and stick to it. If you are in charge of picking up prescriptions for a man who does not live with you—your father or grandfather, an uncle, or a friend, help him establish a relationship with a primary pharmacist, too. Why? Because it is important to have a relationship with the pharmacist and the staff. The pharmacist needs to know who you and the man in your life are. If you go to the same pharmacy, year in and year out, then the pharmacist will get to know a lot about you, beyond simply what doctors and health care providers service your health care needs. If you are developing a relationship with the pharmacist, then he or she can work with your doctor on any questions or concerns. Remember health care should be a team effort.

While it is true that the big chains are mostly computerized and have a record of every script that you and your family fill, computers cannot substitute for human contact with you and the man in your life, and with the doctor who is managing your care. Think back to years gone by when there was an independent pharmacist who was also a businessman or a businesswoman in the community. You were more than just prescription number 42395. You were a person with allergies to milk and peanuts. Your son was a boy with severe asthma. Your father was a type 2 diabetic. And your husband smoked, and had a nasty cough.

The independents are mostly gone, but that doesn't mean that you and your family can't have some of that with the person who works in the chain. But it doesn't happen when you pharmacy hop. And it doesn't happen if you don't talk to the pharmacist or ask questions.

WHAT CAN THE PHARMACIST DO?

The obvious thing the pharmacist can do is fill your prescriptions now and refill them when you run out. The pharmacist is a terrific source of information and can be very helpful for additional concerns. Think about how quick an office visit is. Oftentimes, you don't think of questions to ask regarding medication during the doctor's visit. You can ask your pharmacist those questions. Encourage your man to take notes on the prescriptions that he is getting filled and discuss them with the pharmacist. Or offer to go with him to take notes.

The pharmacist is a teacher of sorts. He or she can be your best source of information on the medicines, what they do, how they work, when they should be taken, and what you should avoid while taking them.

Everybody is looking for ways to save on health care costs. The difference in cost of a generic medicine for, say, high cholesterol, versus the brand version can be as much as $100 or more. If you are filling several prescriptions like this, your pharmacist can help you save several hundred dollars a month, or thousands of dollars over the course of a year, without compromising health effects.

Many of the major pharmaceutical companies have joined forces to put prescription drugs in reach of the uninsured or underinsured. There are several programs such as the Partnership for Prescription Assistance and the Together RX Access program that help those who cannot afford prescriptions. These programs have served lots of people but they are still underutilized.

For more information on the Partnership for Prescription Assistance, including eligibility and prescription drugs covered, go to www.pparx.org, or call 1-888-4PPA-NOW (1-888-477-2669).

To find out about Together RX Access which requires that the person have no prescription drug coverage available to him, go to www.togetherrx.com or call 1-800-444-4106.

Two other great sources of information are RxAssist, www.rxassist.org, and RxHope, www.rxhope.com. Both sites are designed to help health care providers identify resources for their patients, and offer information on free or low cost prescription medications.

WHAT ABOUT BUYING MEDS ONLINE?

Buying your medications online can be a convenience, and can offer substantial cost savings, but buyer beware. Never purchase your medications from a company that will fill prescriptions without a script from the physician. Never drop your desire for quality care in favor of convenience or cost savings. Also remember, some of the savings promised by offshore companies are not real. Many of these companies are being investigated for providing diluted or counterfeit medications. And if you do order your medications from a reputable company, make sure to check them out carefully as soon as they arrive.

GET YOUR MAN A PRESCRIPTION CHECKUP

At least once a year, the man in your life should check with the pharmacist about all the medications he is taking. It would be best to gather them all up (including the nonprescription medications he takes like aspirin or Motrin) in a bag and discuss them with the pharmacist. If he takes everything in, including his vitamins and herbal supplements, the pharmacist can guide him on what should be replaced and what could cause him problems based on the other medicines he's taking.

Timing is everything. There are good times and bad times to do this. Don't expect that the pharmacist will have time to do this with you in peak pharmacy hours when people are lined up around the store. Consider writing down everything your man is taking and leaving the list with the pharmacist. Arrange a time to come back to discuss this with him or her.

GET RID OF THE EXPIRED AND OLD MEDICINES

It is important to get rid of old and expired medications at least twice a year. Expired drugs may lose their effectiveness and potency. Think about doing it in the spring and fall. If you have medications that are expired, call the doctor's office immediately for a refill.

BUILDING YOUR FAMILY MEDICINE CABINET

In addition to the medications that the family physician or specialist recommends, it is a good idea to have your medicine cabinet stocked with certain over-the-counter products. If you have small children at home, make sure everything has a child-proof or child safe cap.

Your medicine cabinet should include the following:

- A pain reliever
- Aspirin
- Antibiotic ointment (reduces risk of infection)
- Antacid (relieves upset stomach)
- Antihistamine (relieves allergy symptoms)
- Syrup of ipecac (induces vomiting)
- Decongestant (relieves stuffy nose and other cold symptoms)
- Fever reducer (adult and child)
- Hydrocortisone (relieves itching and inflammation)
- Antiseptic (helps stop infection)

Questions to Ask the Pharmacist

When you, a family member, or a friend take a prescription to be filled for the first time, there are bound to be questions. Your man may not remember exactly how the doctor or nurse told him to take the medicine. He may have forgotten what the doctor told him not to do, like operate heavy machinery while taking this particular medicine. When he goes to get a prescription filled, urge him to ask any question he has at that time, like:

- Is this the generic form of the medicine? Is the generic just as effective?
- What is the medicine really supposed to do?
- How much of the prescribed medicine should be taken? What happens if I miss a dose at the allotted time? Should I take two to compensate for missing one?
- Should I take the medicine with food or with milk?
- Should the prescription be left in a cool dry place or refrigerator?
- Are there side effects that need to be discussed?
- What should I do if I experience side effects?
- What about over-the-counter medicines? Will my prescription medications interact with these? (Some products like cold medications can raise blood pressure.)
- What effect will the medicine have on sexual performance? (Most men want to know this. In fact, many black men will stop taking their medications for high blood pressure, or other cardiovascular health concerns, if they think they will wreak havoc with their sex lives. This is something that a man should be discussing with his physician. There are many things that can be done for medication-related performance issues.)

WHAT CAN BE DONE AT HOME?

Keeping the medications straight starts at the health care provider's office, but in order for them to do their job, a man must take control when he gets home. He has to understand how and when he is supposed to take the medication. Then take it! Among black men, compliance with doctor's orders on taking medications is very low. It takes the women in their lives to remind them— sometimes often. Learn as much as you can about the medications being prescribed. Utilize reference materials such as the *Physician's Desk Reference*, available at bookstores, or use the online version at www.pdrhealth.com.

Medications should always be kept in their original containers, especially when you are away from home. In the case of an emergency, people will go looking at medications to know what he is taking. If the meds are in their containers, clearly labeled with the dosages, then there will be few questions. Know the expiration dates. Never let him take other people's medications, even if they are yours. Prescriptions are not "one size fits all."

If he is on several medications, use a pill case that lets him set out meds for the week. Some people use little plastic sandwich bags to sort out pills for easy access. He should still keep the bulk of the pills in their original containers.

CHAPTER 5

For the Record

Once you have helped the man in your life settle in with a health care provider, one of the next best things you can do for him, or yourself for that matter, is to keep good health and medical records. Buy two things—a notebook and a set of folders—for each member of your family. You may want to get different colored folders for you and for him. Have them in a place where you can readily get to them, and update them on a regular basis. Keeping good and accurate records can really help with following a preventative or a treatment plan.

WHY USE A NOTEBOOK?

A notebook is an important tool in helping your man manage his health. This is the place where he can write all the questions he has about his health between office visits. It is also the place to write down changes that he notices, or you do, in his health. If he has been having headaches, or is dizzy often, you might want to jot this down so that he doesn't forget to talk about this with his doctor.

Use this notebook to keep all the doctor's offices, phone numbers, and the names of the key office personnel. It comes in handy to be able to call the receptionist, or the nurse who always takes his blood pressure, by name.

The notebook is also a good place to take notes about what happened during the doctors' visits. Many times, important information that needs to be remembered and acted upon will come up in that office visit. A notebook can keep all that information straight. And you will notice that whether you are in the doctor's office or clinic or even at the hospital advocating for a family member's health, when you are writing and taking notes, you get more complete answers from your health team.

When you run out of space in one notebook, don't hesitate to start another. Some people have health notebooks that span decades. They can go back and track what was happening with their health twenty years ago and compare it to where they are today. It may sound like a lot of work but it is worth it.

WHAT DO WE DO WITH THE FOLDERS?

The folders are as important as the notebooks. This is the place you want to keep copies of test results, notes from appointments, a list of your prescriptions and how and when they should be taken. Put up-to-date information on immunizations, tuberculosis tests, childhood diseases, and any other medical conditions in the files. We also put referral notes and health articles of interest in our folders. Make sure to create a section for medical bills and insurance payments. This can sometimes be a maze of information. Your husband or father could easily have a procedure in the emergency room and get six to seven different bills, all from the same health incident. Being able to look at them all in one place will help to sort it all out.

Having the information at hand can help him keep up with his flexible spending account (FSA), if he has one. (An FSA is a tax-advantaged savings account, obtained through an employer, that is used for medical and dependent care expenses.) It also comes in handy at tax time, when you want to take a deduction for health expenses that were not covered by insurance. If you are good at using the computer, you may even want to set up a system, maybe even a spreadsheet, to keep these records on your computer, but for most people it's just easier to keep them in files. Whatever system you use, make it easy.

WHY DO ALL THIS?

While it is true that your family doctor has many of these records (if the man in your life has been going to the same office or clinic for a period of time), there are many reasons why you will want to keep a set of health records at home. Sometimes medical records and test results get lost. The computers that store medical records for large and small health care providers can crash just like the ones you have at home. Health care providers change all the time. The man in your life can easily find himself under the care of several different medical providers in different offices, especially if he needs to be referred to an internist or a specialist, such as a cardiologist. It's always good to have key information available.

HOW DO WE GET THIS?

The first step is to ask the health care provider for a copy of the results of each and every medical test and screening he or she has done. Some doctors instruct the labs to send a copy of the results of blood work directly to the patient. In other cases it has to be requested. Because of the privacy rules, the health care provider will ask your man to sign and return a copy of a form authorizing that provider to release any medical information to you or to be able to talk to you about his health, if he wishes to do this.

He will have to go into the office and fill out a form to make this happen. If he has more than one health care provider, say a family practice physician, an internist, and a urologist, or an allergist, then he should have a set of records for each of them. It's also a good idea to make sure that the offices are sharing information between them. And if he decides to switch doctors, or needs to begin seeing yet another specialist, remind him to make sure that his medical records are shared with the new doctor.

It's so important to get the same kind of information from the pharmacist. He or she should be willing to print out a list of medications, and how they should be taken, for home records. Have your man keep a list of his prescriptions in his wallet, and keep one in your purse, in case of an emergency. We even urge aging parents to make sure that the adult children they call on in a crisis have a list, too.

KNOWING HIS NUMBERS . . .

Throughout this book, you will see some recurring conditions that affect the health of our black men. Hypertension, commonly known as high blood pressure, and high levels of cholesterol can raise his risks for cardiovascular diseases such as heart attacks and stroke. He should be monitored at least once a year by his doctor, and more regularly if he does have high blood pressure or high cholesterol, with an eye to lowering his numbers and managing his health. When he is screened or monitored, make sure that his numbers are recorded in his health records, both in the doctor's office and at home, each and every time.

HIGH BLOOD PRESSURE

One of the biggest risk factors for a heart attack or stroke is elevated blood pressure. In most cases (nearly

95 percent), doctors don't know what specifically is causing it, but in other cases, another underlying illness may be causing the elevated blood pressure, such as kidney disease or a defect in the heart.

Blood pressure is the amount of force exerted through the walls of the arteries as blood passes through them. If there is too much force, it can cause holes or little tears in the arteries. The body tries to heal those tears with clots. If those clots break loose and head toward the brain or block blood going to the brain, it can cause a stroke.

That's why it is so important for the men in your life to monitor their blood pressure regularly, both in the doctor's office and at home, and then take steps to make sure it stays in the normal range.

When taking blood pressure, remember, the top number is the systolic blood pressure and the bottom number, which should always be lower than the top number, is the diastolic blood pressure. The optimum blood pressure is 120/80 or less, but the national median is 129/86. A blood pressure reading of 140/90 or higher is considered high risk.

A man should have his blood pressure taken during every doctor's office visit. It is also a good idea to keep a home blood pressure cuff (measuring tool) at home so that he can monitor himself, especially if he has elevated blood pressure.

HIGH CHOLESTEROL

A high level of total cholesterol in the blood (200 mg/dL or higher) is a major risk factor for heart disease, which raises your risk of stroke. Recent studies show that high levels of *LDL* ("bad") cholesterol (greater than 100 mg/dL) and *triglycerides* (blood fats, 150 mg/dL or higher) increase the risk of stroke in people with previous coronary heart disease, ischemic stroke, or transient ischemic attack (TIA). Low levels (less than 40 mg/dL for men; less than 50 mg/dL for women) of *HDL* ("good") cholesterol also may raise the risk of a stroke. Although there are some hereditary links, many of the causes of elevated cholesterol are found in lifestyle and diet.

Help him make sure he knows and records his most current numbers for ongoing tracking and comparison, as he takes steps to improve or maintain his overall health.

TAKE IT WITH HIM . . .

Having health information in his wallet, or in his PDA, even when he's just going to work or kicking around town can be a lifesaver. Fill out an emergency identification card that will answer key medical questions if he is ever in an accident. Naturally, he will not be able to answer pertinent questions if he is unconscious. This card is sometimes offered by insurance companies, but can also be purchased from your pharmacy. Having this little card with his vital information, such as who to contact, personal doctor, blood type, allergies—especially to anesthesia—most current blood pressure numbers, diabetic status, types of medications, and how to reach you, can be critical.

Another thing to consider is the importance of taking medical information, and a backup plan for lost prescriptions, when you travel.

FAMILY HEALTH HISTORY . . .

When a man goes to a new doctor, the office staff almost always asks him, as a new patient, to fill out a medical history form. It asks basic questions that give the doctor and the office staff a snapshot of his overall health. The form asks questions about tests he has had and the last time he had them, and goes through a list of health conditions that may be affecting him. Sometime during that first visit he may also be asked about his family health history.

Family health history provides insight into a man's risk for certain kinds of diseases. There are many diseases that run in families, such as diabetes and certain kinds of cancer. Some of it is hereditary or as the new buzz calls it "genetic," and some other factors may be at play, like family health and lifestyle culture. Because people of color have never done a lot of talking about their health, very few know the whole picture of what illnesses parents, siblings, and grandparents had.

We never openly talk about a family member's depression or suicide. We don't talk about sexual dysfunction, or substance abuse and how it affects our health. A man may know that his father died of a heart attack at age forty-five, or that his sisters all had breast cancer, but he may not know enough of the details to have a complete picture of his health history, both genetic and cultural. The information is scattered, at best.

That's why there is a new push for families to get together and explore their family health histories. The more information a person has about his health history and his risk factors, the more he can work to prevent history from repeating itself. History and risk factors are just that. By making important lifestyle changes, staying on top of early detection screenings, and taking necessary medication, we can reduce our risks for many illnesses. But it is important to know as much as possible about our risks.

Where to Start

Very few black men take the time to seek out key health history information on their own. Some families have started looking at their health history as a part of their work in studying their family trees.

Summer picnics, reunions, and other gatherings are perfect times to pull out those old photo albums and share long-forgotten family stories. But they are also perfect times to gather your family's health history—and it may even save your life. Tracking your family's medical history can help identify health risks that run in families and help you chart a plan of action to stay healthy for years to come.

By taking the time when you are with family, you can get a more complete and accurate picture of your family health history. Just by asking the questions, you may be able to find out that there is a family history of certain chronic diseases.

With more talk about the importance of genetics, and the DNA tests being done to find out what our real roots are, there is a better understanding of the importance of history.

A recent study done by the Centers for Disease Control shows that 96 percent of the people they surveyed understood the importance of family health history in maintaining overall wellness and health literacy. The study also shows that less than a third of those surveyed had actually taken steps to gather and document this information. The biggest reason for the gap? Most people don't know where to start or what questions to ask when it comes to tracking their family health history.

It's not all in the genes, according to medical experts. We forget about the lifestyle and culture that impact our family health history. Some scientists believe that indeed there are hereditary links to chronic diseases that are triggered by obesity, such as diabetes and high blood pressure, but they also know that diet and the amount you and your family exercise play a major role.

If your family eats large portions of a high fat diet and has little physical activity, then this may be the biggest historical influence in your family's incidence of diabetes and heart disease. A man may have several incidences of deaths from colorectal cancer in his family, but it may or may not have anything to do with genetics. It could be that his family has never eaten much of a preventative diet of fruits, vegetables, and whole grains. Maybe no one in his family has ever had any of the early screening tests for the disease, and they were diagnosed when it was too late for treatment.

Genetics and history tell a part of the story, but we can make significant lifestyle changes that can impact our lives and our futures.

The Office of the United States Surgeon General, the National Institutes of Health, the Centers for Disease Control and Prevention (CDC), the Agency for Healthcare Research and Quality (AHRQ), and the Health Resources and Services Administration (HRSA) have come together to develop an easy-to-use family health history form—the My Family Health Portrait—that can be downloaded from the Internet to help you gather your family's information. The form asks for information about the health and illnesses of both sides of a person's family. The form also allows for modification to address more customized information. It can be used right online and saved only to your computer to protect your family's privacy. But if you'd rather have a hard copy, it is available for free by going to www.hhs.gov/familyhistory/order.html or order a free copy by mail at 1-800-ASK HRSA. Mayo Clinic's Web site, www.mayoclinic.com, also gives comprehensive information on how to compile family health history.

Put your family health history to work. You may do a great job over the coming year of gathering all your family health history information and sharing it, but you need to put it to work. And make sure you update it regularly.

Chart a Plan of Action

If your detective work uncovers a family history of a particular illness, use it as an opportunity to talk to the men in your life about what you found and how together you can reduce the risks for illnesses, complications, and death. Encourage them to talk to their doctors about creating a prevention plan of action. Together you may decide that it is time to make serious changes in your lifestyle or diet. Your risks for certain disease may trigger the need for more regular screening and diagnostic tests to catch disease earlier.

Privacy

The whole subject of genetics and use of testing has raised fears that your health history can be used to jeopardize your employment or ability to get and maintain health insurance. As of April 2003, individuals in all fifty states have medical privacy protection under the Health Insurance Portability and Privacy Act (HIPPA). Most states also have medical privacy information laws, as well. While many genetic counselors say that the risk of having your family health history used against you is minimal, you should make sure you ask important questions about how the information will be used, and if the results of tests will be made available to your insurers or employers. For more information on privacy and medical records as covered by HIPPA, check out the nonprofit Privacy Rights Clearinghouse's Web site, www.privacyrights.org.

Do It for the Children

By taking the steps now to uncover and understand health history, you can make it easier for future generations to do a lot better. You may find that your search for family health information is not always easy. It may require hunting down birth and death certificates, going through the old family Bible, and seeking other information. Keep great medical records to pass on to your children.

Tips on How to Build Your Family Health History

- Download the Family Health History program from www.hhs.gov/familyhistory and print out the forms.
- Explain to your family members why you are doing this and how you will use the information. Offer to make your report available to them for their use, as well.
- Pay close attention to immediate family history first. Did his father have a heart attack? Did either of his parents or his siblings have colorectal cancer?
- Look at both sides of his family tree. Don't just assume that you should look only at his father's family for links to information. Both sides can hold equally valuable health cues.
- Pay attention to everything. A family health history of breast cancer among his sisters and his mother may not seem very relevant, but it is. Men don't get breast cancer with the frequency that women do, but it does

happen. Plus, as a man's daughters and future generations look at their health risks, it becomes increasingly important that he is able to pass that information down from both his mother's and father's family trees.

- Get information on the age when a person was diagnosed with an illness. A family history of men who have had heart attacks under age fifty raises many risk red flags for the other men in a family.

- Talk to as many family members as possible to get a complete family history profile. Go beyond his siblings and parents, if you can. You may see links to cousins, aunts, and uncles who are also living with the same family risks.

- Look at family birth and death certificates to help you piece your family health history puzzle together.

- Get the next generation involved. Make it a family project so that the next generation begins to understand the importance of health and wellness.

What Should You Do with the Information?

Family health history is an important tool that should be used by all families of color. A family health history that is never put to good use in helping to make changes is as useless as one that is never taken at all. So do it and use it.

- Encourage him to take his family health history report to his physician, so that it can be added to his medical records.

- Sit down together and have an honest discussion on what the health risks really mean to the two of you. Discuss what your individual risk factors are for key diseases, such as cardiovascular disease, diabetes, certain cancers, and Alzheimer's, with your physician, based on your family health history.
- Work closely with him and his doctor to develop a strategy for prevention and early detection of diseases. Use the clues that his family health history gives to maintain good health. If the people in his family who have suffered strokes ate a high-fat diet, or were inactive, then make a plan to help him to start moving.
- Encourage other family members (parents, siblings, and cousins) to use the information to get regular testing for diseases that put them at high risk for certain diseases.
- Keep the family health history momentum going. Share the information with your sons and daughters so that they can become aware of their own health risks and take action.

BUILDING A SUPPORT SYSTEM

If it takes one village to raise a child, it takes many of villages to keep us healthy. No matter how independent a man feels he is, he can benefit from a strong support system of family, friends, and co-workers. Sometimes as we struggle with health issues, it is that support system that keeps checking in, giving encouragement, attending doctor's visits, and just being prepared to listen sometimes that is invaluable.

Help the men in your life understand the importance of building a health support team. The chances are great that most of the people in that support system are people that are a part of his circle of friends and family, anyway. But because men tend not to talk about their health concerns in any direct way, your man probably has not called on his circle to lend this kind of support. Now is the time to do it.

The family needs to be at the core of the support system for any man, and have a real understanding of what is being asked of them and why. Also think about a support system that includes other men. It really does help to have someone who has something in common with you to discuss and answer questions on a health crisis, or in prevention. If your man is struggling with his weight, his support system might include a friend who has lost weight and kept it off, to talk about how he did it. Maybe his friend also needs to lose weight and get fit. Together they may come up with a game plan to start moving.

Don't forget that women need support in this journey, too. Build your support system of other women whom you can talk to about developing positive solutions to health prevention challenges with the men in your lives. Say, you still can't get your dad to go to the doctor to have a prostate screening. Maybe you and the sister-friends you are close to in your place of worship decide that all the men need to be screened. Then plan a screening evening at the church. That's a way that support can work. Try creating "no junk food" or no smoking zones at your homes and supporting each other in that effort. The point is to work together and be creative on behalf of our men.

The Health Buddy

Another very valuable person in his health support team is a health buddy. All adults, no matter what their age or gender, should have one, especially our black men. This is the person who might go to the doctor with him. He or she takes notes, to make sure what was said is what was understood in the office visit. A health buddy checks in to find out if the man has filled his prescriptions and is taking his medicines, and if there are any questions that really need to be answered. He or she is the extra set of ears and eyes when it comes to health.

The health buddy is also a real health advocate. If a man is hospitalized and in pain, you can help him by being his health buddy, the person who can talk to the doctor or hospital staff on his behalf, to see if the pain can be managed better.

In many homes, husbands and wives are health buddies for each other, but it could be anyone. The point is to identify that person before a health crisis. Ask if he or she is willing to act in that role, share what the expectations of everybody are, and then get to work.

Sharon Davis is her big brother's keeper. She and her sister Karen Williams call and check in on their big brother John Williams once a week. But on one particular call, Sharon says, "He sounded different." She couldn't put her finger on what she was picking up in this call, but somehow he sounded not quite like himself. "We even asked him about his health, but he said he was fine," she says of John, who has been in good health all his life. She says there was no one thing or set of things that concerned her. Her instincts just told her that something wasn't right. "I told him that I thought he needed a checkup, but he seemed to be dragging his feet," she says.

Digging around a bit, Sharon found out that one of the problems was that her brother did not have a health care provider with whom he felt comfortable. Sharon says they contacted three doctors before they found one who would take him and his borderline high blood pressure seriously. "My brother is a gentle, quiet man. He didn't feel that the doctors were really listening to him and seeing him." Sharon wanted answers, so she got in the car and drove eighty miles to go to his appointments with him.

"Now that he has great care, he manages his health care well on his own," she says. His high blood pressure is under control, he is working to maintain a healthy weight, and he is doing fine—thanks to a sister who would not take no for an answer.

As we talk about the biggest killers of black men— heart attacks and complications from a stroke—you will see that we will keep talking about the role of high blood pressure and elevated cholesterol and weight control, because they are crucial to health and wellness. Even though people of color may have a predisposition to higher blood pressure levels than their white counterparts, these levels can be controlled through diet, exercise, relaxation techniques, and medications.

Having a support system in place and running can help your black man reduce his weight, lower his cholesterol, and reduce his risk of heart disease. Think about the big Sunday dinners, or family gatherings. These get-togethers are a huge tradition in families of color, but they may not be very healthy as far as diet goes. Before you switch everybody over to nuts and berries, take some time to build support for making modifications in meals that will probably make everyone healthier. Talk about portion control. Share recipes that still taste awesome, but are lower in cholesterol-raising ingredients. Maybe as a family, you decide to limit the amount of alcohol served at family gatherings. The point is that building a family support system doesn't just work for the man in your life. It can help build healthy habits and a new sense of wellness for everyone.

The Role of Spiritual Community in Support

Spirituality is a key part of the culture and essence of black America. Our places of worship have been the glue that held us together when nothing else would. They are institutions that are still the hubs of our communities. As people become more spread out in cities and around the country, the church is playing an even more important role in keeping us connected. If you want to find some black people and create connections, go to your church or worship place of choice.

Our religious communities have the power and sheer numbers to have a major impact on the health of black people in their congregations. We are seeing health ministries grow within the churches and mosques. Groups are sponsoring prostate screenings, blood pressure days, and even exercise programs to make the community healthier. As much that is going on, we urge you to do more. There is no illness that black people suffer from that health outreach and education can't impact. The best place, outside of the home, is probably the place where we worship.

Mrs. Vivian Berryhill is the president of the association that represents the wives of the black ministers in the country. She says there are so many issues that the churches are asked to address. "Our church communities are being asked to deal with health, but they are also addressing poverty, homelessness, the education of our children, and building networks for services for our seniors," Mrs. Berryhill states.

As Mrs. Berryhill says, many faith-based organizations are coming together to close gaps and give access around the health of our communities. The Metro Denver Black Church Initiative is expanding its partnerships through the Center for African-American Health. They are hands-on in the community with a focus on reducing the serious health disparities that affect black people living in the Metro Denver area, for example. They use community-based health education, research, and outreach that promote active and healthy lifestyle behavior. The program has been able to provide culturally appropriate health education and screening to over 15,000 black men and women in Denver each year.

The National Cancer Institute (NCI) is getting the message of the power of faith and spirituality in reaching out to communities of color. They are linking up with the faith community around the country to encourage black men and women to eat a healthy diet as part of an active lifestyle. The program, called Body and Soul, offers the black faith community a guide and training materials to help them incorporate these activities into programs that already exist. The American Cancer Society is also having great success nationwide in creating outreach and support in black communities through its Body and Soul program.

African Americans Reach and Teach Health (AARTH) is another impressive faith-based program out of Seattle that is trying to respond to HIV/AIDS and other major health issues affecting people of African descent. Reverend Mary Diggs-Hobson, Reginald Diggs, and Dr. DeMaurice Moses wanted to work with churches, mosques, and other faith-based and community organizations to bridge the gap in health disparities by providing health education and training, and this program is their solution.

These programs and many others—new and already flourishing around the country—are important in sending messages about black men's health and keeping them front and center. Together we need to support these programs and create them where they don't exist. With our faith and fellowship, we can move mountains.

CHAPTER 6

Obesity

There are so many health problems that we as black women need to help the men in our lives address. It is hard for us to know where to start. Start at the beginning. Obesity and being overweight are major problems for both black men and black women. Ask any medical professional and he or she will tell you that if you could reduce the numbers of overweight or obese men of color in this country, you would also be able to impact almost every illness that leads to early death, with the exception of HIV-infection and lung cancer.

Being overweight, having a poor diet, and not getting enough exercise increase a black man's risk for high blood pressure, heart disease, stroke, many cancers—including colorectal, pancreatic, and prostate cancer—diabetes, arthritis, and depression. It is no coincidence that black men have an extremely high incidence of all these diseases.

WHAT IS OBESITY . . . REALLY?

According to the Office of the United States Surgeon General, 300,000 deaths of both men and women in this country are linked to obesity each year. Being overweight or obese is caused by consuming more calories than are needed and a lack of physical activity.

The Body Mass Index (BMI) is a mathematical calculation used to determine whether a person is overweight or obese. Being obese and being overweight are not the same condition. A person who is considered overweight has a body mass index between 25 and 29.9. An obese person has a body mass index over 30. A man can be overweight without being considered obese. Both put the body at risk for chronic disease.

BMI is calculated by dividing a person's body weight in kilograms by his height in meters squared (weight [kg] / height [m]^2) or by using the conversion with pounds (lbs) and inches (in) squared as shown below.

This number can be misleading, however, for very muscular people, because BMI does not measure body fat. Two men with the same height and weight can have the same BMI even though one person may be very athletic (a bodybuilder, as an example) and the other may be shorter and overweight. So it is a good idea for the man in your life to discuss this with his health care provider to determine his overall health risk factors. But if you want to try it at home, here is how you can calculate his BMI:

$$[\text{Weight (lbs)} / \text{height (in)}^2] \times 703 = \text{BMI}$$

Again, a man with a BMI of 30 or more is considered
obese and a BMI between 25 and 29.9 is considered
overweight. Another example is a man who is 245
pounds, and is 5 foot 10 inches, who has a body mass
index of 35.2. The number of men and women of color
who are overweight and obese is growing and this is affecting their overall health and wellness. Table 6.1 shows
that black people in the United States are becoming
more overweight and more obese over time.

Table 6.1
**INCREASE IN OVERWEIGHT AND OBESITY PREVALENCE
AMONG U.S. ADULTS* BY RACIAL / ETHNIC GROUP***

Racial / Ethnic Group	Overweight (BMI ≥ 25) Prevalence (%)		Obesity (BMI ≥ 30) Prevalence (%)	
	1988 to 1994	1999 to 2000	1988 to 1994	1999 to 2000
Black (non-Hispanic)	62.5	69.6	30.2	39.9
Mexican American	67.4	73.4	28.4	34.4
White (non-Hispanic)	52.6	62.3	21.2	28.7

SOURCE: CDC, National Center for Health Statistics, National Health and Nutrition
Examination Survey. Flegal et. al. *JAMA*. 2002; 288:1723–7 and *IJO*, 1998;22:39–47.

*Ages 20 and older for 1999 to 2000 and ages 20 to 74 for 1988 to 1994.

WHY OUR MEN NEED OUR HELP

Black folks carry a lot of baggage. As you will see in almost ever chapter in this book, it is hard for them to seek out help and support. Unlike alcoholism or mental health issues, being overweight carries its own baggage. It is not viewed as a disease, but a sign of weakness. "If you just pulled yourself away from the table, you wouldn't be fat," is what a lot of people say.

There are many reasons why people become overweight or obese. But the most common answer is that we are taking in more calories than we burn or use as energy. Metabolism is the process that turns the food we eat into energy. The human body needs energy to do its work. It uses energy from caloric intake for breathing, circulating blood throughout the body, growth and repair of cells, each and every day. We also use energy to digest our food. We use much of our energy in physical activity, such as walking around the block, or playing basketball or football. While many attribute their weight gain to a slow metabolism, or their slim physique to a more rapid metabolism, experts at the Mayo Clinic say that most of the cases of weight gain that lead to being overweight or obese are due to an imbalance of calorie intake to use of energy. Again, we eat more than we burn through physical activity. But as we all know old habits die hard.

Food is so deeply rooted in black culture. Most black men, especially if they were born in the United States, were raised on high fat foods and lots of them. And we all know that the words "portion control" have been virtually non-existent in our vocabulary until recently.

Food represents love and care. Being able to eat whatever you want whenever you want is a type of affluence, even when nothing else exists. Somebody wants to show you that they care, so they bake you a coconut cake. If you want to show your appreciation for a meal, you have to heap your plate high, and then come back for seconds. When someone dies, even if they died of an obesity-related disease like diabetes, friends and neighbors show their support by bringing truckloads of food around. Yes, ladies, we have a lot of work to do to reshape those cultural messages to make our men, and ourselves, healthier.

HOW DID OUR MEN
GET THIS WAY?

If he's not paying attention and taking precautions, it is easy for him to slowly gain weight. Ladies, this is something we have known about ourselves for years. But did you know that a man over thirty usually gains over a pound and a half every year? This gain happens because men eat the same amounts of food in their thirties, forties, and fifties and are often less active than they were in their twenties. As we said, being overweight or obese is caused by taking in more calories than your body can use. Black men (and women) are eating more and exercising less—a surefire recipe for being overweight or obese.

Many black men drive everywhere. He may be making poor food choices when he's left to his own devices. He could be drinking high-calorie alcoholic beverages. And he may be spending hours in front of the television to unwind. He doesn't even have to get up to walk to the television to change the channel, thanks to remote controls.

Yes, it is true that some of us may be genetically pre-disposed to being overweight, but our genes do not have to dictate the end result. Scientists at the National In-stitutes of Health who are looking at family health history and genetics suggest that culture should be factored into the role that family health history plays.

As an example, if your man comes from a family of overweight or obese people, maybe it is not all in the genes. It may be that he comes from a family that eats huge portions of high-fat, high-sugar foods, and rarely exercises. It is more likely that each family member's choices in the amounts and types of food he eats, and how much physical activity he chooses to do, are the biggest factors in how well he is able to control his weight.

Maybe it has to do with the high-fat-content foods, like fried chicken and pies, that are a part of his family rituals and the family food rituals you are building in your own home. When shopping for food that will help break the cycle, remember that not all fats are created equal. Although there are things such as good and bad fats, monosaturated fats, such as animal products, are the ones that should be reduced or used in moderation.

Perhaps the huge portions that were served in the family have played a role. Maybe that combined with the lack of exercise within a family has resulted in a family history of obesity. These are hard, often generational, habits to break, but with your help he can do it.

WHAT CAN WE DO?

If we want our men to be healthier and live in a state of wellness, instead of chronic ailments and disease, we have to help them make lifestyle changes. We live in a fast-food, on-the-run nation. Although some restaurants are offering healthier options on their menus, much of the fast food that is served is contributing to our nation's obesity. Sugar-heavy sodas, fries, shakes, and burgers are not the best food choices to build a diet around. Delivery pizza may be convenient for the busy family, but it is not a good foundation for a healthy diet.

Consider the importance of preparing more meals at home. Even though it seems to take more time, you have more control over what is eaten. You know if the food is prepared in fat or oil. You know if there is enough fiber in the menu and if it is balanced and nutritious. If you are cooking at home, you have much more control over the amount of salt that is going into the diet of a person who is monitoring his high blood pressure. In fact, many people who have had great success losing weight and keeping it off have reduced the amount of meals they have outside the home, and have learned to make very careful food choices when ordering in restaurants and in carryouts.

In many households, the woman of the house is the primary grocery shopper. She is also usually the primary decision maker on what gets served in the house. In planning your meals, you need to have a good understanding of what is considered nutritious, balanced, and healthy.

We have to re-educate ourselves and the men in our

lives as to what is a healthy diet. If you live in the house with a meat-and-potatoes man, you know how challenging this can be. But remember that the diet of meat-and-potatoes can impact a man's risk of heart disease, diabetes, stroke, and cancer.

For decades the United States Department of Agriculture has had something called a food pyramid, which helps define what a person needs each day to maintain a healthy and balanced diet. The food pyramid suggests that the dietary guidelines for a healthy diet include whole grains, fat-free and low-fat milk and dairy products, lean meats, chicken, and fish. It also suggests that men eat five servings of fruits and vegetables a day.

The food pyramid recommends the following daily servings:

- Strive for 2–3 servings of dairy, including milk, yogurt, and cheeses, such as an eight-ounce glass of milk, or a yogurt smoothie.
- No more than 2–3 servings of meats, poultry, fish, dried beans, eggs, and nuts. A meat serving is about 2–3 ounces, or the size of a deck of cards.
- Between 6 and 11 servings of grains per day. A serving is one slice of bread, or one-half cup of rice.
- Eat 3–5 servings of vegetables in a day. One serving is a cup of raw vegetables or one-half cup of cooked vegetables.
- Consume 2–4 servings of fruit per day. One serving is one-half cup of cooked, chopped, or canned fruit or one medium-size apple. Three-quarters of a cup of fruit juice is also considered a serving.
- The National Cancer Institute takes that advice even

further by recommending that men, especially men of color, eat even more fruits and vegetables than are recommended in the food pyramid. They are suggesting that men eat at least 9 servings a day of fruits and vegetables. It may seem challenging to get all these servings in. But it's not, if you are creative.

Planning healthy, balanced meals in advance helps to avoid the "I don't know what to cook, so I'll order out" trap. Get a slow cooker. You can quickly put together a healthy meal that will simmer all day. By the time you get home from work, dinner is served. Or try cooking several meals on the weekend, when things are not so hectic, and freezing them for dinners during the week. Think meals that can be popped in the microwave or oven.

When you are looking for new recipes or planning your meals, reduce or eliminate fried foods, or foods prepared in butter, heavy creams, and sauces. Substitute a seven-day-a-week diet of meat and potatoes for a baked, grilled, steamed, or poached fish like fresh tuna and wild salmon—which offers more heart-healthy protection than farm-raised—at least two days a week.

Prepare more fruits and vegetables—with caution. Don't ruin a healthy food choice like fresh greens or green beans with greasy salt pork or other grease-laden meats. And don't overcook them. Vegetables that are lightly cooked offer a wonderful source of dietary fiber.

Cut back on salt. Learn more about adding flavor by adding onion, garlic, fresh and dried herbs, lemon, and other natural seasonings. Salt use can elevate blood pressure. Replace the saltshaker on the table with alternatives like Mrs. Dash, or a good old bottle of Tabasco.

Encourage everyone to taste the food before reaching for the saltshaker.

What Should He Eat?

If you want to make an impact on the health and well-being of your loved ones, the best place to start is in the kitchen.

- Consume no more than 30 percent of daily calories from fats of any kind.
- Watch the portion size.
- Eat more fish, but find creative ways to cook it. Cut way back on fried foods, even chicken or fish.
- Get dairy into the diet, but go with low-fat products like skim milk, low-fat yogurts, and low-fat cheeses.
- Make a habit of having salads with lunch or dinner. They are a wonderful way to help the man in your life meet the goal of nine servings of fruit and vegetables a day. Also experiment with steamed and grilled vegetables. Add plant protein like peanuts, and other nuts.
- Eat whole-grain cereal with skim or low-fat milk and fresh fruit.
- Serve beans. They are a terrific source of protein and fiber. Cook them as a side dish or sprinkle them in salads.
- Shake the salt.
- Make sure he's getting enough whole grains that are found in some breads, brown rice, and whole grain pasta.

By now you are thinking that if you make these changes, he won't eat it. He'll just stop eating at home. The truth is that you both may need to retrain your taste buds, but this little step could be a lifesaver in the long run. And if you are creative with the seasonings you use and the way you prepare the food, you may not miss the old way at all.

Recently, Kenda Tibbs, a registered dietician, catered a lunch for a large meeting of black men and women who came together to discuss health disparities and cancer prevention. Kenda served up a soul food lunch, complete with smothered chicken, green beans, black-eyed peas, dressing, and hot homemade rolls. Some attendees complained about the meal because they felt that a health luncheon should be, well, it should be healthy. They said this as they licked their fingers and went back to the buffet table for more.

Imagine their surprise when Kenda announced that every single item she served was within the recommendations of the American Cancer Society, the American Dietetic Association, and the American Heart Association. She baked the chicken, instead of serving it fried. She used more seasonings and less salt, she used smoked turkey in her green beans, and as she says, "I never cook them to death." She even served a healthy peach cobbler. "It takes a good cookbook and some creativity, that's all," Kenda says. (Table 6.2 offers easy substitutes for bad food choices.)

Get rid of the soft drinks that are high in sugar. One little can of soda may not seem like a lot, but it is loaded with sugar, and over time can help pack on the pounds. And research shows that on average, each American is

Table 6.2

EASY WAYS TO SUBSTITUTE HEALTHIER FOOD CHOICES

Subtract	Add In
White breads	Whole grain breads
Salt	Seasonings to layer flavor like garlic, peppers, and onions
Sugary sodas and juice drinks	Water, tea (easy on the sugar)
Fried chicken	Roasted or baked chicken
Fried fish	Steamed, baked, or grilled fish such as wild salmon
Cooking with heavy grease and animal products like salt pork	Sauté in olive oil, or canola oil
Bottled salad dressings	Olive oil and vinegar dressings
Cake or pie for dessert	Fresh fruit for dessert
Whole milk	Skim milk
Hard liquor or cocktails	A glass of wine or a wine spritzer
Ice cream	Low fat yogurt with fresh fruit
Candy or chips	No salt or lightly salted peanuts or other nuts, if he doesn't have nut allergies

drinking 53 gallons of soft drinks a year. Did you know that a large Coke at a fast-food restaurant is 32 ounces and contains 310 calories? Or that a 12-ounce can of soda contains 10 teaspoons of sugar and 140 to 150 calories. So if a man is drinking three to four cans of soda a day, he's taking in as much as 600 of his calories in soda pop.

Start weaning him off the soda, to help him maintain a healthy weight. Keep cold bottled water around the house as an alternative to sodas. The body is primarily made up of water. It keeps the body hydrated, especially if you are active. It also aids in the digestive process. By slowly reducing high-calorie drinks and replacing them with the recommended 8 eight-ounce glasses of water or more, he will start to see some of the weight come off.

GET HIM MOVING . . .

Encourage him to be more physically active. It does not mean that he has to become a gym rat or a competitive bodybuilder. Subtle changes can make a big difference. Encourage him to take up some of the activities he loved to do when he was younger, like golf. Get a gym membership, and encourage him to go (you could go too). But remember, never let your man start any kind of exercise routine without clearing it with his health care provider. Your doctor can be your best ally in convincing him to make significant lifestyle changes.

Beginning to become more physically active does not mean going from being a couch potato to a marathon man. Slow and steady is probably the best course. It not only gets the body adjusted to its new lifestyle, but will also help prevent injuries that can sideline him.

Walking is a terrific way to become physically active. Take evening walks after meals, or get a treadmill and put it right in front of the television if you have to. But treadmills aren't really necessary. Walking is essentially free. Many people start their new exercise and physical activity routine by just walking for ten minutes each day. Then they work up by adding a couple of minutes, or a couple of minutes at a faster rate each week. Encourage him to get his time up to at least thirty minutes a day.

Nina Moore, a certified personal trainer in Los Angeles, who works with athletes and celebrities, says that thirty minutes is a good start, but likes to see her clients work their way up to forty-five minutes of cardioaerobic activity like walking or running and add in some strength training like weights. She also says that it is important to take a few minutes before and after a workout to stretch those muscles. "Warming up and cooling down is very important," Nina says. She also encourages men to include exercise into their regular routines for increased physical activity.

Here are a few suggestions:

- Park the car farther away from the store or office and walk.
- Take up a new activity like tennis or swimming.
- Pass on the golf cart and walk the nine or eighteen holes.
- Take the steps instead of the elevator or escalator.

- Spend more time working in the yard; it's a great way to work up a sweat.

LITTLE EFFORTS YIELD BIG RESULTS . . .

It always seems that our men have an easier time losing weight than we do, if they put their minds to it. There are many reasons, including the fact that muscle burns fat, and men tend to have more muscle mass than women. And don't forget that because men need more calories than women to just do the basics of walking and sitting, as well as physical exercise, they burn calories faster. But they still have to work hard at it if they want to lose weight.

If he is overweight or obese, your man may have to stay at it a while to reach his goals, but even a small weight loss can yield big results in improving a man's health. Just think about it—a 10 percent weight loss, or say 25 pounds in a 250-pound man, can reduce his high blood pressure and high cholesterol numbers, as well as relieve some of his heartburn symptoms. Weight loss will help him breathe easier and relieve some of the pressure that can cause chronic knee and other joint pain.

There are 3,500 calories in a pound of fat. So if a man expends 3,500 calories more than he takes in, through a food deficit or using more calories in physical activity, or some combination of the two, he will lose one pound of weight.

Many of us watched television each week to see Pete

Thomas, a property investment manager, beat the battle of the bulge the old-fashioned way—sort of. He entered the *Biggest Loser* challenge as the heaviest of the competitors at 401 pounds. Although he did not win the overall competition, because he was voted off, he really was the biggest loser of all the competitors. He lost 185 pounds (83 during the show competition and another 102 at home) and over 46 percent of his body weight through grueling exercise and dramatic modification of his diet. Pete's story is inspiring on many levels including the fact that his wife Pam took on the challenge at home and lost 76 pounds herself.

"While Pete was away, I was determined that he wasn't going to come home new and improved, while I was still overweight. So I started cutting out fried foods and watching my portions, and I lost weight," Pam says.

But she also had to step up her game when Pete came home. He had more weight that he wanted to lose and she was instrumental in supporting him in his goal. "I took the lessons he learned on the show about cooking healthier, portion control, and how to eat out and rolled them into our everyday life." She also got aggressive about working out with him, six days a week. "We are partners in this," she says.

Thanks to that teamwork, Pete was able to get his blood pressure back to normal and eliminate the joint pain and difficulty moving and walking. He is an overall healthier and happier person. Together they have made a commitment to support each other in staying healthy and fit for the rest of their lives.

Where many of us struggle with the scale fairly privately, America's top weatherman, Al Roker, dealt with his weight issues every day in front of the camera at the *Today* show. Over the last three years, Al lost over 100 pounds after opting to have high-risk gastric bypass surgery.

Al and his wife, ABC news correspondent Deborah Roberts, are careful to tell anyone who asks that such a radical procedure is not the magic bullet. It is expensive and often is not covered by insurance. The national average cost is about $26,000.

No one should take on this type of surgery lightly. There is a 1-in-200 death rate for those who opt to have the procedure. Al says that he was reluctant to go public with having the procedure done because he never wanted to be thought of as an advocate or a role model for gastric bypass. He and Deborah agree that it was a tough decision, but one that was right for them. "I didn't want him to do it for me," Deborah says. "He had to want to do it for himself. And he did."

Gastric bypass, for men like Al, is only the beginning—a jump start. Al has had to significantly alter his diet and change his lifestyle. But he stays on track, thanks to Deborah's *gentle* encouragement. "I still have to coax him off the couch to get moving," she says of Al, who works out optimally five days a week with his trainer. "I'm a health fanatic. I work out three days a week with a trainer and take some classes, so it's hard for him to put one over on me."

"Sometimes he might think I am nagging, but I'll take that," Deborah says. "That's what I need to do to keep him healthy and around for me and our children."

She also pays close attention to his diet, which is not easy. Al's struggles with food would seem to be complicated by the fact that he is a bona fide food lover. With his cookbooks, and television shows for the Food Network, it's never easy. Al states people have told him that it seems like making an alcoholic a bartender. "You're doing these cooking shows. You do these cookbooks. But the fact is unlike alcoholism, you can live, you can survive without taking a drink. You got to eat," Al says.

Edwin Crump is not a nationally known public figure, but he too opted to have the surgery two years ago. "My wife, Georgann, and I talked to a lot of people, and did a lot of Internet research," he says of the preparation they did before making the decision. "I had sleep apnea that was affecting my heart and blood pressure. I was having the beginning of type 2 diabetes," Edwin reports.

"I had been worried about Edwin's health for a long time," Georgann says. "But it was ultimately his decision. My job was to support him every step of the way."

They also feel that the surgery was just a jump start. "I overhauled everything I do. I don't eat pork anymore. I use a sugar substitute. I lay off the sweets. And I work out," says Edwin. He was over 400 pounds when he started his journey, and has lost 150 pounds and is still losing weight. "I feel better. I was able to give up all of my medications for hypertension, diabetes, and high cholesterol," he says. "I feel like I got my life back."

EMOTIONAL EATING

Believe it or not, we women are not the only ones who grab the ice cream when we are upset or anxious. Our men are doing it, too. Many of the men we talked to said that in addition to just loving good food, they grabbed the food at times of stress, boredom, sadness, depression, or anxiousness. And unfortunately our black men don't tend to grab the celery sticks or grapes when they are under pressure. Most people know what their food triggers are. They also tend to grab the same kinds of foods, each time they need to feed the emotional dragon.

Al Roker says that one of the big changes for him was that he couldn't use food as a crutch anymore. He has worked hard to look within for the answers. "The surgery doesn't change what's in your head," Al says. "You have to look at what's triggering the overeating and deal with it."

Radio superstar Tom Joyner has said that he had times when he was also an emotional eater. The Fly Jock struggled with his weight when he was logging in thousands of miles a year flying back and forth from Chicago to Dallas every day. He works hard to keep weight off, says his wife, fitness guru Donna Richardson.

"Tom is just a big guy," Donna says, of her husband. "People see him and don't understand that he lost forty pounds and is keeping it off." She says that his workout plan and weight loss have brought his blood pressure down and lowered his health risks. Donna says she motivates him, but she says he has found his own motivation to stay on track in feeling better and being able to keep up the pace he needs to "keep being the Fly jock."

But Donna, who is helping thousands of men and women get moving through her Sweating in the Spirit program of diet and exercise, says she leaves the day-to-day of helping Tom up to him. "He has his own trainer and his own chef."

Each day is a new day. It's never too late to get back on the right track. If the man in your life slips up and gives in to emotional eating, work with him to get back in the groove of eating well and mindfully.

Tips for Controlling Emotional Eating

Black men and black women both can be prone to using food as a crutch or stress reliever. It is one of those old habits that is bad, but it dies hard. Here are some tips for getting a grip on the emotional eating that packs the pounds on:

- Try to eat only when hungry and don't skip meals. Skipping meals can lead to overeating.
- Remove the unhealthy junk foods from the house. These are the first foods we go for when we are looking for a little comfort.
- Replace the bad snacks with fruit or raw vegetables like carrots.
- Stay away from alcohol when feeling emotional. The high-sugar/high-calorie content of alcohol can blow a diet.
- Get lots of rest. People tend to overeat when they are feeling tired.

- Make sure that meals that are eaten are balanced. And pay attention to portion sizes.
- Make exercise a part of the daily routine, especially in times of stress. Yoga, walking, running, and other physical activity can help.

WHAT ABOUT OUR BOYS?

Childhood obesity is an epidemic. Data show that a child who is obese or overweight is more likely to struggle through life as an obese adult. Doctors are treating children with chronic health problems like type 2 diabetes, high blood pressure, and joint pain—things that they used to see only in overweight adults. According to the Centers for Disease Control's Youth Risk Assessment Survey of high school students from grades 9 through 12, 16 percent of all high school students are considered obese or overweight. The survey shows that more black students (22 percent) are considered overweight or obese than their fellow white students (14 percent), putting them at higher long-term risk for the chronic diseases we have been talking about.

There are many reasons, but the formula is pretty much the same. All of our children are eating bigger portions, higher fat and sugar foods, and getting less physical activity. The safety nets that our boys used to have, such as gym classes, outdoor recess, and a variety of sports that were free, have been reduced or eliminated.

It's not just limited to African American communities. These issues seem to play a bigger role in urban areas. As do factors such as shortages of places for families to buy fresh, wholesome foods, information about healthy, balanced meals and their importance, and safe places to walk, play, and exercise. We also have to recognize the role that culture plays in self-image. While black teens are less likely to give in to the pressures that society puts on them to be super thin, and to develop eating disorders, they are also more likely to develop complications from being overweight or obese.

As we discussed earlier, America has become a convenience society when it comes to our diet, and unfortunately we are passing that down to our children. Where it used to be a special treat for a child to get food that was not cooked at home, data shows we are now living on fast food, which is helping to make our children overweight. Busy families find it easier to go through the drive-through window at the fast-food restaurant, or order a pizza, so that there is food on the table. Limit the number of times that your family eats fast food a week. Sit down together for family meals whenever possible. As children's schedules get busier, this becomes more difficult. It requires commitment and planning.

If you want your children to do better you have to teach them how. Take your children grocery shopping with you and show them how to make healthy choices. Explain why an apple is better for him than a candy bar. Stress the importance of drinking milk (soy milk if the child is allergic to dairy products).

Teach them that the French fry is not a key part of a nutritious food group. Ask them how specific foods fit

into the food pyramid. And take it to the next step by in-
volving him in food preparation at meal time. Use
cooking as a teachable moment. Many of us have some
of our fondest family moments around food and
cooking. Not only is it tradition, but a once-in-a-lifetime
opportunity to build healthy families.

Even though parents have control somewhat of their
children's eating at home, it takes a lot more work to get
the junk out of their diets at school. The school vending
machines, which are a big moneymaker for struggling
school districts, are loaded with high-sugar-content soft
drinks that offer no nutritional value. Many of our
children consider a balanced lunch meal a bag of salty
chips, a candy bar, and a soda. If black women want to
make an impact on the health and well-being of their
children and get rid of bad habits before they start, they
have to work on what their children are eating at school.
Send them to school with healthy snacks. Make sure
they have access to milk and bottled water. Pack their
lunches with healthy foods.

And work with your school administration on what
foods they are serving the children for breakfast and
lunch. Be an advocate for the children in your community
by insisting on healthy food choices in the schools.

As parents and communities who want to carve out a
better future for our children, we have to address one of
the biggest culprits in the childhood obesity story, the
lack of exercise. We are creating a generation of couch and
computer potatoes. We have to get then moving again.

There are several ways to encourage your sons to be
more active. Limit the amount of time your child spends
in front of the television or video game. Children who

spend a great deal of time doing such things are less likely to be physically active and more likely to be overweight or obese.

Obtain a family membership to the YMCA if you can afford it. Don't just send them, go with them. Use the time at the Y as quality family time, swimming, playing basketball, and staying active—together. Use the great outdoors—it's free. Take family walks. Invite other families to play softball or tag football. Break out the Rollerblades or the bikes. Take advantage of the facilities that are available through the parks and recreation programs or Boys and Girls Clubs in your town.

TIPS . . .

Here is a recap to help the men and boys in your life become fit and shake some of the weight that is making them sick and increasing their health risks:

- Have the conversation. You can't decide to make him lose weight without his cooperation. It is something he must want to do and see the value in. Tell him that it's not about appearance, it's about living longer and stronger. Everybody who loves him also needs him around.
- Set up an appointment for him to talk to his doctor and get the "all clear" before he starts a workout routine.
- Learn how to substitute healthy cooking methods for some of the less healthy ones, such as frying or cooking vegetables in fat.

- Take the saltshaker off the table.
- Offer more water and less soda and alcohol.
- Preplan to avoid the need to run to the drive-through at the end of the day.
- Take the pizza parlor's number off your phone's speed-dial.
- Help him make an exercise plan that he can live with.
- Serve meals at the table and not in front of the television.
- Get him to eat his last meal of the day at least two hours before he goes to bed. Encourage him to cut out middle-of-the-night snacking.
- Pack healthy snacks for him to keep in the car or put in his golf or gym bag.
- Go out dancing together.
- Load the refrigerator and freezer with healthy meals he can pop in the oven or microwave on days you aren't home.

CHAPTER 7

Cardiovascular Diseases

As of 2005, it is estimated that 70 million Americans have some form of cardiovascular disease. Cardiovascular disease is not limited to heart disease. The cardiovascular system includes the heart, but it also includes the veins, arteries, and capillaries that carry blood throughout the whole body, including the lungs, kidneys, and brain.

Heart attack and stroke account for the majority of cardiovascular disease and make up 40 percent of all deaths of men and women in this country. Most heart attacks and strokes could have been prevented through lifestyle modification such as exercise, stress reduction, weight loss, screening, and complying with treatment for high blood pressure and high cholesterol (for more information see chapter 5, For the Record). In this chapter we will take a look at heart disease, heart attacks, strokes and aneurysms, and deep vein thrombosis. These are major cardiovascular diseases that are taking a toll on our black men and our community.

HEART DISEASE

Heart disease, which is a condition that negatively affects the heart muscle or the veins and arteries that lead to and from the heart, is a major problem for both black men and women. Heart disease is the leading cause of death of black men of all ages. But black women's numbers of heart disease are actually higher than those of our black men. Our communities lose thousands of black men and women prematurely because of heart disease and fatal heart attacks.

The medical community has been wrestling with all the reasons why for decades. But the one thing we do know is that diet, lack of exercise, and uncontrolled cholesterol and blood pressure all contribute to a black man's risk for heart disease, because they can damage, clog, or eventually completely block the arteries that pump blood to and from the heart. And unfortunately, it isn't unusual for black men (or women) to have many of these risk factors that put their hearts in jeopardy.

Why Is the Heart So Important?

This might sound like a silly question, but when you look at the way so many of us, including our men, take care of our hearts, it's pretty clear that people don't really understand the heart's importance.

The heart is a muscle. But it is the most important muscle in the body. It pumps blood and oxygen to and from other parts of the body, including the brain. It is the centerpiece of what is known as the cardiovascular system. As you know, without a functioning heart, a person would die. And with a heart that is not working the way it should, the man in your life could be experiencing shortness of breath, dizziness, or inability to be mobile for long periods of time—symptoms of underlying heart disease. Left undiagnosed and untreated they could lead to a minor, or massive, heart attack.

What Are the Risk Factors for Heart Disease?

- Age—The older a man gets, the more his risks increase.
- Gender—More men get heart disease but women's numbers are growing.
- Heredity
- High blood pressure, high cholesterol, diabetes
- Being overweight or obese
- Being African American
- Excessive alcohol intake
- Tobacco use
- Uncontrolled stress
- Eating a high-fat diet

What Causes a Heart Attack?

A heart attack is the result of restricted blood flow to and from the heart. This happens when the arteries that send blood to and from the heart narrow from plaque buildup, clogs, and clots that will ultimately restrict all flow to the heart and cause a heart attack.

Emmett Spears, a seventy-eight-year-old husband, father, and grandfather from New York, appeared to be the picture of health. He ran to stay in shape, but owned and managed a high-pressure business for more than forty years. Little by little, he was experiencing warning signs that something was not right. "I was running a business. I couldn't afford to be sick. Nobody wants to do business with a sick person," Emmett says.

It was only after he had a heart attack that he knew he was going to have to take major steps; he put it off for as long as possible. He had heart surgery for a blockage and got a heart stent that keeps the arteries open. After again experiencing a loss of energy and some chest discomfort, he went in for tests, which showed another major blockage. In 2005 he had a second heart surgery to replace his stent with a new one. His daughter, Angela Spears Rochester, who lives in Denver, says her dad had done what men do. "He just kept going. And then he had a full-blown heart attack, of all places, on the subway in New York."

Emmett made a full recovery and continues to lead an active life by walking several miles a day, but it taught him a serious lesson about self-care. "I just eat chicken and fish until I'm sick of it. But I do it," he says. He has given up using oils and fats, including butter. "The hardest thing to give up was bacon, lettuce, and tomato sandwiches, but I gave that up, too," he says.

Angela says that her father's heart condition has taught her own husband, Mark, a few lessons about diet and exercise. Together Angela and Mark decided to take the steps to be healthier by cutting out unhealthy snacks and being more active. She says that she has changed the way she eats, but for Mark, it is a work in progress. They both have made the commitment to a healthier lifestyle in order to keep up with their young son, Aidan.

What Does a Heart Attack Feel Like?

One symptom can be a sharp pain in the chest. Other symptoms may be more subtle and easier to ignore. They tend to start slowly, with just a little mild pain. And although few people talk about some of the other symptoms, pain or numbness in the arms, or sharp pain in the back, neck, or jaw can also be signs that a person is having a heart attack. Shortness of breath in combination with chest pain, cold sweats, nausea, and vomiting or dizziness can all signal a heart attack. An actual heart attack can last several minutes. But because there is often damage that goes with the attack, a person can have abnormal heartbeats, called arrhythmias, that can last for several hours or even days after, like the aftershocks of an earthquake.

If there is any question that your man might be having a heart attack, it is vital to get him immediate medical attention. A person having a heart attack that is treated within the first four to six hours is more likely to survive the attack.

The Warning Signs of a Heart Attack

Although some people have minor heart attacks, without any warning signs, most have one or more of these symptoms:

- Chest pain
- Chest pressure that feels like "an elephant sitting on the chest" or someone squeezing the heart
- Discomfort or numbness in arm, jaw, back, or stomach
- Shortness of breath
- Dizziness
- Nausea
- Cold sweats

Get Thee to a Doctor . . .

Don't let him play doctor with his heart. One of the biggest mistakes that our men make is that they ignore the warning signs of a heart attack. They assume they have heartburn. Many men gamble by thinking they can just shake it off. And indeed, they may be able to momentarily shake it off, but they could be causing permanent damage to their hearts. It's a gamble they can't win. Many people never have symptoms, but later find out that they have had several little heart attacks and never even knew it. Unfortunately, when those people have "the big one" it usually is really big, and often fatal. So don't wait for the subtle symptoms to get worse. Heart attacks require emergency treatment.

Be Prepared

If you don't know cardiopulmonary resuscitation (CPR), take a class. It could mean the difference between life and death for someone you love. By taking a little time to learn proper CPR skills today, you may be taking a step that could save someone you love tomorrow. While it is absolutely crucial to call 911 or get a person who may be experiencing warning signs to care, it is also important to keep that person alive until help arrives. The American Red Cross teaches lifesaving CPR techniques all around the country. So do many hospitals and health care facilities.

Encourage your workplace to purchase a defibrillator, which is a computerized device that measures heart rhythm and recognizes when the heart needs a shock. It does this through voice prompts to the person using it. In the case of a cardiac emergency it could be all that stands between life and death for you or your co-workers.

Don't Second Guess It . . .

If he complains of any of these warning signals, call 911 right away. Be as calm as possible. Be prepared to clearly tell the person on the phone what is going on and where the Emergency Medical System workers can find you. You can always drive the person to the hospital yourself, but the American Heart Association says that patients who come to the hospital in an ambulance and are experiencing chest pains are usually getting faster treatment than ones who are brought in by car. The staff is not only trained to get a man to the hospital, they are also trained to revive him if his heart has stopped.

Heart Disease Is Preventable

Black men do not have to be written off as statistics. The women in their lives can help reduce their risks by supporting them in managing their weight loss, blood pressure, and cholesterol; maintaining a healthy diet; giving up smoking; and getting some exercise. We can use the information that is out there about making diet and lifestyle changes, medications, and stress reduction to help them keep their hearts healthy for many years to come. Don't wait until the man in your life hits middle age and beyond to start making changes. Our young children are already developing habits such as inactivity and a diet of high-sugar, high-fat foods that will put them at great risk twenty, thirty, or forty years down the road.

We also know that heart disease in communities of color is not an old man's disease. Our young men are showing signs of blocked arteries and shortness of breath at earlier ages than ever before. In fact black men between the ages of thirty-five and forty-four have twice the death rate from heart disease that white men in that age group have.

Atlanta's first black mayor, Maynard Jackson, had a heart attack that proved to be fatal in 2003 while walking through the airport in Washington, D.C. He had struggled with heart disease and obesity, and in 1992 he had bypass surgery for six blocked arteries.

Broadcaster Ed Bradley had been suffering with what he thought was acid reflux to later find out that he had major blockages in the main artery of his heart. He had lifesaving quintuple bypass surgery. But he is one of the lucky ones.

One of the things you are going to hear from us over and over again is prevention. As mothers, daughters, sisters, and wives, we have the potential to make a huge difference in helping our men prevent a heart attack or cardiovascular disease.

Here are some tips on heart disease prevention:

- Insist that he get a yearly physical, even if you have to make the appointment. He should have his blood pressure monitored and a blood test that measures his cholesterol levels as a part of this physical.
- Help him quit smoking. Smoking not only increases his risk for lung cancer, but it also can clog his arteries and put him at higher risk for a heart attack. Did you know that 70 percent of heart attack patients are smokers!?
- Support him in maintaining healthy blood pressure and cholesterol levels. Take the salt off the table. Too much salt can raise blood pressure. Consider serving a little wine with dinner. Studies show that drinking a glass of wine once a day can help lower blood pressure. Moderation is the key.

- Cook more fish (not fried or loaded with sauce). Start shopping for fresh wild salmon and other cold water fish such as trout, tuna, sardines; they offer not only healthy proteins, but are rich in omega-3 fatty acids that can help keep the arteries clear. These are better choices than eating saturated fatty meats. Shoot for two to three times a week. Also don't forget introducing a fish oil tablet into his daily supplements.
- Have him ask his doctor about adding a low dose or baby aspirin every day. Low-dose aspirin has been shown to reduce clotting and clumping in the blood that can narrow a blood vessel and cause a heart attack.
- If you are cooking for him, reduce the bad things and add in the good. Cut back the fatty and processed foods. Get rid of saturated fats and go for healthier monosaturated fats that help to control cholesterol, and weight. Add in more fruits and vegetables.
- If he lives in a cold winter climate, make sure he is careful about exerting himself while shoveling snow.
- Tell him to get moving. He needs at least thirty minutes of cardiovascular exercise a day, once he gets the okay from his doctor.

Getting Screened and Diagnosed for Heart Disease

Screening and diagnosis are important in the fight to reduce the risk of death from heart disease. It is important that men of color are regularly screened for high blood pressure, high cholesterol, and C-reactive proteins, which are indicators of high risk for heart disease.

Studies such as *Unequal Treatment: Confronting Racial and Ethnic Disparities in Health Care,* from the Institute of Medicine, show that there can be unequal care in the health care system between black men and their white counterparts when it comes to diagnosis and treatment for heart disease and heart attacks. The studies show that black men who come into the emergency room with symptoms that could mean a heart attack are not always offered the same state-of-the-art tests and treatments as white males. Data from the Institute of Medicine show that black men are less likely to have lifesaving angioplasty and cardiac bypass surgery than white males. The drugs that are being developed for heart disease and stroke may not be as effective in black men and women, because they are not being developed for or tested on people of color.

Be prepared to insist on screening and diagnostic tests that will rule out heart disease before an event occurs. And if he does have a heart health crisis that requires emergency medical attention, be vigilant in asking questions on next steps and appropriate treatments. Unfortunately black men and women are less likely to get those tests. They are more likely than white males to get sent home from the emergency room without diagnosis or treatment, especially if they have no insurance.

According to a report released by the Leonard Davis Institute at the University of Pennsylvania, geography also plays a role in the cardiac care that black patients receive. The report says that some of these disparities exist because many black patients live in areas where health technology of all kinds, including the latest developments in cardiac care, are available but are underutilized.

There are several ways that doctors determine the existence of heart disease or if a person has had or is having a heart attack. These are not normally given as routine screening tests, but when there is a strong suspicion that there is heart disease or a heart attack.

Electrocardiogram

The electrocardiogram is the most basic form of a heart diagnostic tool. Sensors are attached to the chest and the electrical impulses that regulate the way the heart pumps blood are measured. If there are any abnormal patterns in the readout they can signal that all is not right with the heart. An abnormal EKG usually leads to other tests.

Stress Tests

The stress test is used to evaluate the heart and vascular system during exercise. It helps answer two general questions: Is there underlying heart disease that only becomes apparent when the heart is stressed by exercise? And if there is underlying heart disease, how severe is it? The patient is attached to an ECG machine, and a blood pressure cuff is placed on one arm. Sometimes a clothespin-like sensor is attached to the finger to measure the amount of oxygen in the blood.

After a baseline ECG is taken, the patient begins to perform a low level of exercise, either by walking on a treadmill or pedaling a stationary bicycle. The exercise is "graded"—that is, every three minutes, the level of exercise is increased. At each "stage" of exercise, the pulse, blood pressure, and ECG are recorded, along with any symptoms the patient may be experiencing.

Cardiac Angiogram

An angiogram allows doctors to view the condition of arteries. Doctors insert a catheter into the artery in the leg and move it up through to the heart. They then send a dye through the catheter that shows the arteries under an X-ray. A blockage that shows up on the angiogram could be restricting the flow of blood and cause a heart attack.

CT and PET Scans

These are diagnostic tests that give doctors a view of the arteries without doing any invasive procedures. A person who is getting a CT scan does get an injection of dye to highlight the blood vessels and show calcium buildup, as well as fat-filled plaques and blockages in the arteries. Overweight people may not be good candidates for a CT scan because excessive body fat can distort readings.

Positron emission tomography, also called PET imaging or a PET scan, is a diagnostic test that takes "pictures" of the heart based on radiation. Magnetic resonance imaging (MRI), and echocardiograms, which are ultrasounds of the heart, have proven useful in diagnosing heart disease.

Treatment for Heart Attacks

Treatments for heart attack can vary based on the reason for the blockage or heart attack and its severity. Some heart attacks can be treated with medicines while others are treated with surgery. It is in the best interest of the man in your life to research the options. Ask a lot of questions on his behalf about why a health care provider is suggesting one treatment option over another. You want to ask questions about the severity of the heart attack and the likelihood of reoccurrence with each of the options.

The most common heart attack treatments are discussed next.

Coronary Artery Bypass Surgery

A surgeon will take a blood vessel from another part of the body, usually another spot in the chest or in the leg and make a "bypass" away from the blocked part of the artery. You may have heard of double or triple bypasses. This happens when there is a blockage in more than one spot and it becomes necessary to create *several* of these bypasses.

A bypass surgery is a major surgery. It is never done on an outpatient basis. You should expect that without any complications he should be in the hospital for three to five days. Also be aware that it will take some time for him to get back on his feet after this kind of surgery. It is not uncommon for a man to suffer surgery-related depression and memory loss while he is recuperating.

Angioplasty

This procedure is used to diagnose heart disease, and find and treat blockages. A cardiologist will use a catheter with a balloon attached to it. The balloon is inflated to move the plaque and clots away to make room for blood to flow properly. This is not usually a complicated procedure. A man will usually be asked to stay overnight for observation and then be released.

In addition, he may be given medications by his cardiologist and monitored carefully. Alpha- or beta-blocker medications are given to almost all men who have heart attacks, after the incident, whether they have surgery or not.

Medications

- *ACE inhibitors.* The ACE inhibitors, such as Capoten, Lotensin, and Vasotec, work to reduce a substance in the blood that can cause vessels in the blood to tighten and elevate blood pressure. The ACE inhibitors are given to a heart attack patient to lower blood pressure and to make it easier for the heart to do its work while it is recovering from the attack.
- *Calcium channel blockers.* Calcium channel blocker medications such as Cardizem, Procaroia, and Vascor, keep the arteries open by blocking out calcium that can enter and clog the arteries. They also work to slow down the heart so that it can work more effectively.
- *Cholesterol-reducing medications.* He may already be on these medications that are designed to lower cholesterol. He may get a new prescription for these to

lower the bad cholesterol, in order to protect him from some of the things that caused the heart attack in the first place.

• *Aspirin.* Yes, the little aspirin pill that you have had in the medicine cabinet all this time. The medical community now sees this as a wonderful way to keep both heart attacks and strokes away. Aspirin keeps platelets from clotting and clogging the arteries. Cardiologists suggest that chewing an aspirin during a heart episode can reduce its severity and maybe save a life. It doesn't take a lot of aspirin to do the trick. A chewable baby aspirin once a day can work to prevent a heart attack.

If a man is over forty, and has a history of high cholesterol and or high blood pressure, ask his doctor if aspirin therapy might be safe and beneficial for him.

STROKE

Without question Luther Vandross was one of the premier singers and performers of our time. We all watched him struggle with weight and other health issues, including diabetes, for years. His mother, Mary Ida Vandross, and other women who loved him and were closest to him say that the ups and downs of his weight, high blood pressure, high cholesterol, and the stress took its toll on him. The price he paid was a massive stroke in 2004.

Patti LaBelle, who herself has struggled with her weight, diabetes, and other health issues publicly, loved Luther. She was a part of his support system before the stroke and during his efforts at rehabilitation. "What happened to Luther should be a wake-up call for all of us," she says. "We have to take better care of ourselves if we want to be here."

Luther was a black man who seemed to belong not just to his mother and to his friends, but to all of us. And when the news got out that Luther had had a stroke, we all prayed. Occasionally we would get glimpses of him trying to rebound and come back to us. But it was not to be. Even though we knew he was not doing well, the country was stunned when it was announced that he had died. We still have his music, but we all wish he was still here making songs that make us laugh and cry and fall in love all over again.

Although Luther had incomparable talent, fame, and a large support system, in the end he was another black man whose body failed him. His story set a cautionary tale for both black men and black women. "If it could happen to Luther with all his resources, then maybe I should pay attention," we all said. But old habits die hard. And we never really think what happened to Luther Vandross could happen to us. But it does every single day.

What Is a Stroke?

A stroke occurs because of damage to the arteries that lead to the brain. It differs from other cardiovascular diseases that affect the arteries and veins that transport blood to and from the heart, and the heart itself. Strokes are the third leading cause of death in this country. Statistics show that 150,000 to 160,000 people will die of a stroke this year, and unfortunately, many of them will be black men.

Strokes most commonly occur when the blood supply to the brain becomes blocked in some way. Over 80 percent of strokes are due to a blood clot. The other strokes occur when a person is suffering with an undiagnosed "leaky" blood vessel that builds internal pressure in the brain.

The American Stroke Association commissioned a Harris Poll to learn more about how much we, as people of color, know about our health risks for stroke. The findings were bleak. Although 70 percent of the black men and black women they interviewed said they knew what a stroke was, only 30 percent could correctly define a stroke. The poll revealed that only 49 percent said they knew how to recognize stroke symptoms. Most startling, over half of the people they talked to mistakenly thought they were at no risk for a stroke. But we can turn the tide on our knowledge of prevention of stroke by educating ourselves and our families.

Symptoms and Warning Signals of a Stroke

Some say that stroke is a silent killer. But in reality, the silence is due to the fact that men will ignore or shake off the warning signs their bodies are giving them. If a man is experiencing numbness or tingling, especially on one side of his body, difficulty talking or understanding when other people are talking, suddenly having trouble seeing or walking, or dizziness, then he could be experiencing a stroke. Others report having what they call the worst headache they have ever experienced, prior to having a stroke. Sometimes the symptoms will come and go.

Timing Is Everything . . .

If you even think that there is a chance that someone might be having a stroke, call 911 or another emergency medical service immediately. The golden three minutes after a stroke, and the care a person receives in those key minutes, can mean the difference between life and death.

Help Him Reduce His Risks

One of the best ways to prevent strokes is to reduce the risk factors that can cause them. Many factors can contribute to a person having a life-threatening stroke. No surprise, but the more risk factors the man in your life has, the more likely he is to be vulnerable to a stroke. And also there is no surprise in the fact that the risk factors for a stroke are the same as some of the risk factors for heart attacks. A man who is obese or has diabetes, high blood pressure, or high cholesterol has an increased chance of having a heart attack or stroke.

Velma Henderson, chief nursing officer at Howard University Hospital in Washington, D.C., sees hundreds of black men come into the hospital who have had strokes. "Black Americans are now suffering from strokes earlier in life and dying more from strokes than whites," she says.

In 2006, sports fans were shocked when baseball star Kirby Puckett died from a stroke at age forty-five. It was yet another wake-up call for black men who think they have all the time in the world to take their health and well-being for granted.

Transient Ischemic Attacks (TIAs)

TIAs are "warning strokes" that produce stroke-like symptoms, such as numbness and or tingling in the face, arm, or leg, usually on one side of the body, and confusion, trouble seeing, and difficulty speaking. They do not last as long as a stroke and generally don't cause lasting damage. Because initially, it is very difficult for a person without medical training to tell the difference between a TIA and a stroke, it is important to call 911 to receive medical help immediately. Recognizing and treating TIAs can reduce the risk of a major stroke. Nearly one-third of people who have a TIA will have a stroke later, if the causes of the attack are not treated— either through medication or surgery, or a combination of the two.

Atrial Fibrillation

This heart rhythm disorder raises the risk for stroke. The heart's upper chambers quiver instead of beating effectively, which can cause the blood to pool and clot. If a clot breaks off, enters the bloodstream, and lodges in an artery leading to the brain, a stroke results. Symptoms include chest pain and having a hard time catching breath at the smallest exertion.

People with coronary heart disease or heart failure have a higher risk of stroke than those with hearts that work normally. Dilated cardiomyopathy (an enlarged heart), heart valve disease, and some types of congenital heart defects also raise the risk of stroke.

Other Risk Factors

There are many other illnesses, conditions, and lifestyle choices that can put a person at high risk for a stroke. Knowing the risks and taking the right steps to reduce them can help to prevent a stroke.

• *A high red blood cell count.* An elevated red blood cell count thickens the blood and makes clots more likely. This raises the risk of stroke. Doctors may treat this problem by removing blood cells or prescribing "blood thinners." It is important to have a red blood cell count as part of routine blood work during the visit to the doctor or health care provider. A healthy man should have complete blood work done at least once a year.
• *Excessive alcohol.* Drinking an average of two drinks a day for men can raise blood pressure and may increase risk for stroke.
• *Some illegal drugs.* Intravenous drug abuse carries a high risk of stroke because it can damage the vessels

that supply blood to the brain. Cocaine use has been linked to strokes and heart attacks. Some have been fatal even in first-time users.

• *Smoking.* Tobacco use seems to have an extremely damaging effect on a person's cardiovascular system. Experts say that the nicotine and carbon monoxide in tobacco smoke can reduce the amount of oxygen in the blood that goes to the brain. Tobacco smoke also damages the walls of the blood vessels to the brain, making it easier for the clots that cause strokes to form.

Unavoidable Risk Factors

In addition to the points listed above, there are some other things he can do to reduce his risk of stroke: Make lifestyle changes, such as eating a healthy and balanced diet, reducing stress, and being physically active. If he is on medication to control his blood pressure, it is important that he be diligent about taking it as prescribed. However, there are some risk factors that come with the package:

• *Increasing age.* People of all ages, including children, have strokes. But the older you are, the greater your risk for stroke. Black men over forty are at higher risk.

• *Sex (gender).* Stroke is more common in men than in women. In most age groups, more men than women will have a stroke in a given year. However, women account for more than half of all stroke deaths.

• *Heredity (family history) and race.* Your stroke risk is greater if a parent, grandparent, sister, or brother has had a stroke. African Americans have a much higher risk of death from a stroke than Caucasians do. This is partly because blacks have higher risks of high blood pressure, diabetes, and obesity.

• *Prior stroke or heart attack.* Someone who has had a stroke is at much higher risk of having another one. If you've had a heart attack, you're at higher risk of having a stroke, too.

• *Sickle cell disease (also called sickle cell anemia).* This genetic disorder mainly affects black Americans. "Sickled" red blood cells are less able to carry oxygen to the body's tissues and organs. They also tend to stick to blood vessel walls, which can block arteries to the brain and cause a stroke. Unfortunately, stroke occurs most commonly in infants and children who have sickle cell disease. Knowing your genetic status is key to preventing the birth of a child with sickle cell disease and therefore the possibility of having strokes that begin in infancy.

What Can I Do to Help Him Prevent a Stroke?

You can help him by reminding him to take his meds. The medical community agrees that one of the biggest risk factors for stroke is failure to take medicines that control high blood pressure and cholesterol. Sometimes men stop taking the medications for high blood pressure and high cholesterol because they don't want to feel dependent on medication or are experiencing side effects like being overly tired or constant thirst. Stopping these medications can put a man at great risk for a heart attack or stroke.

After the Stroke

Walter Conyers suffered a stroke in 1997. Ten years later, he says he is still getting better every day, but it took a lot of work. "People don't understand what it's like. How scary it is," he says. Walter initially lost use of the right side of his body (which is common in stroke victims). While he did not have to have surgery to restore his mobility, he had to re-learn how to use those muscles and re-learn to speak through extensive physical and speech therapy. "I had a hard time with the most common words. Anything that began with an *S* or an *STR* gave me a fit," he says. Having a good rehabilitation therapist helped, but he also says the support and under-standing of the people in his life, including his co-workers, was invaluable.

"It definitely changed my life," he says. "Before the stroke, I was quite a debater. I would argue labor disputes on my job, and could out-talk anybody." But he says that the stroke left him having to work hard to gain those skills back. Many men have difficulty after a stroke, including diminished use of the arm or leg on one side of the body. They may also have difficulty re-gaining their speech or their cognitive thinking skills. Physical, occupational, and speech therapy can be im-portant components in helping a man recuperate after suffering a stroke. It is important for the women in men's lives to support and gently urge men in their efforts to go through therapy and rehabilitation.

The Invisible Man

Robert Harris, like Walter, is a man who is fighting to return to where he was before his stroke. He's back at work in his job as a supervisor in an automobile plant, but still struggling to gain full use of his speech. He is blessed to have the unending support of his longtime companion, Dorothy.

"I keep pushing him at times when he would rather give up. I make him get out and be around people when he would rather stay home and hibernate," she says. Rehab experts say that after a stroke socialization is very important for a man to get back on his feet.

"The speech thing has been difficult for him to accept," Dorothy adds. But it has also been difficult for people around him. Both Robert and Walter talk about the feeling of invisibility while trying to recuperate. "People feel uncomfortable. They don't know whether to talk to me or talk around me. They don't know whether to give me eye contact or to look away," Robert says. Walter agrees that this is a hard part of recuperation from a stroke.

They both acknowledge that as strong, independent black men, dealing with the aftermath of a stroke, or any debilitating illness, puts their worst fears of dependence right in their faces. "I never wanted to be taken care of," Walter says. "People had to take care of me, because I could no longer do it myself. Men don't like to talk about being afraid or being scared, but that scared me."

As the nurturers, women have a tremendous role to play in helping the man in our lives recuperate from a stroke. We need to remember that he is still the same man. We also need to be aware that his dignity, self-image, view of his livelihood and manhood, as well as his role in the community, are all wrapped up in his fight to bounce back. It takes patience and love to help usher him back to a normal life.

Preventing strokes in the first place is crucial to our community, but we should not forget about the supporting role we must play in helping a black man get back on his feet after a stroke and preventing recurrences. A person who has had a stroke is more likely to have a second stroke within the first five years without due diligence.

The American Stroke Association offers a terrific resource for people recovering from a stroke and their families, called Stroke Connection. Sign up online for your free subscription at www.strokeassociation.org.

CEREBRAL ANEURYSM

You may be familiar with a stroke, but may not know the difference between a stroke and a cerebral aneurysm. A cerebral aneurysm is the dilation, bulging, or ballooning out of part of the wall of a vein or artery in the brain. Cerebral aneurysms can occur at any age, although they are more common in adults than in children and are slightly more common in women than in men. They can occur without warning signs.

The signs and symptoms of an unruptured cerebral aneurysm will partly depend on its size and rate of growth. For example, a small, unchanging aneurysm will generally produce no symptoms, whereas a larger aneurysm that is steadily growing may produce symptoms such as loss of feeling in the face or problems with the eyes.

Immediately before an aneurysm ruptures, an individual may experience such symptoms as a sudden and unusually severe headache, nausea, vision impairment, vomiting, and loss of consciousness. If you suspect a person has had an aneurysm or a stroke, call 911 right away. Every minute is vital.

Heart attacks and strokes are not the only cardiovascular diseases that can threaten a life.

DEEP VEIN THROMBOSIS

You might not know what deep vein thrombosis (DVT) is, but as a black woman who loves and cares about a black man, you should. It is one of those silent, but preventable killers that we just don't know much about. Yet the complications from deep vein thrombosis kill more than 200,000 Americans each year. According to the Coalition to Prevent Deep-Vein Thrombosis, more people suffer from DVT in a year than heart attack and stroke.

Black men are at high risk for DVT, just as they are for many diseases that affect their hearts and cardiovascular systems. If he already has some kind of heart or respiratory disease, a man's risk can go up even higher. DVT is actually more common than most of us know.

What Is Deep Vein Thrombosis?

Deep vein thrombosis is a very serious condition. It happens when a blood clot forms in a deep vein, usually in the legs. A common complication of DVT is a pulmonary embolism, which happens when a part of the blood clot breaks away from the vein and travels up to the lungs and can actually block the pulmonary arteries in the lungs. Although you may have never heard of DVT, it is one of the leading causes of death in this country. Two million Americans have some form of DVT each year. Many people who develop a pulmonary embolism can die in a matter of hours if left untreated.

Even if a person does not have a pulmonary embolism, DVT is still very dangerous. It can cause chronic swelling and pain in the legs, feet, and ankles, and can damage the blood vessels in the legs. It can make a difference in the quality of life for a man.

A rapid heart rate, shortness of breath, and chest pain are common symptoms of DVT. If he is experiencing these symptoms, a man must seek medical attention right away. Once he is at the hospital or doctor's office, his health care team can begin to diagnose and treat him right away.

How Is a DVT Diagnosed?

There are many ways that doctors diagnose DVT, but the most common one is a venous ultrasound done on the skin of the leg. The ultrasound can detect blood clots in the veins that may be slowing or blocking the flow of blood.

Jim Howlett is a renaissance man. He works shifts in an automobile plant. He spends his spare time in bookstores—reading newspapers, people watching, and holding court with other book lovers. When we asked Jim, who is now single, but has been married twice, if he has ever had a woman in his life guide him through a health crisis, he got a twinkle in his eye. "My daughter, Miriam, saved my life," Jim says. "I could have died from deep vein thrombosis."

Jim continues: "I was at work, and she showed up at my job, because she just had a feeling. She was in college several hours away and she missed classes just to come and insist that I go get checked out." Miriam knew that Jim had had a bout with DVT once before. She got him to a doctor, who examined Jim and confirmed that he was experiencing DVT.

"I needed to be in the hospital right away, just like my daughter said." Jim says he was prepared to drive himself to the hospital, but the doctor had him transported by the medical van immediately. "She was right," Jim says. "And if she hadn't come to my job and insisted, who knows what would have happened. I could be dead."

Traveler's Thrombosis

Some people refer to the type of deep vein thrombosis that happens when people take an airplane flight as traveler's thrombosis, or economy class thrombosis. But it can occur in anyone who is sitting for long stretches at a time, including people who work for hours at a desk. So if he is taking a long flight or is going to be sitting for a period of time, help him reduce his risks by reminding him to . . .

- Take 161 milligrams of aspirin (two baby aspirins) before a long flight to help make the platelets in the blood less sticky and prone to forming clots.
- Wear special support socks during travel, or while working at his desk for hours.
- Get up and walk around the cabin or stretch his legs in the aisles, when the seat belt signs are turned off.
- Walk around and stretch every twenty minutes or so while sitting at a desk.
- Drink plenty of water, which will also keep him hydrated during the flight.
- Wear loose-fitting clothes.

How Is DVT Treated?

The traditional methods for treating diagnosed DVT are elevating the affected leg, getting plenty of bed rest, wearing pressure socks, and taking blood-thinning drugs—such as Coumadin or heparin—to prevent life-threatening clots.

CHAPTER 8

Diabetes

For us, the poster man for this book is a man named Chris Dunbar. When he first heard that we were writing a book specifically for black women on how to help black men take charge of their health, he told us it was a silly idea. Chris came to Andrea at a party, with his wife, Reitu Mabokela, in tow, to tell her that the idea was off base. "I take great care of my own health," Chris said. "She doesn't need to take care of me. I stay on top of it."

He said it with such conviction, but Andrea sensed that there was more to the story. She looked at Reitu, who was standing behind Chris. Reitu gave her "the smile." Ladies, you know the smile we give each other when we have decided to just let him have his say. It's the "I'll tell you about it later" smile.

Chris is a smart, funny, insightful man with a gentle

spirit. Because of the hundreds of health interviews Andrea had done over the years, she knew that he probably had taken control of his health, but she also knew from doing these interviews another truth. She leaned in and got eye level with him and said, "I bet you've had a significant health incident." Well you should have seen the look of surprise on his face. It was true. Chris had been diagnosed with diabetes not long before he met and married Reitu.

The diagnosis began to change the way Chris approached his health. But he keeps moving in the right direction thanks again to the gentle guidance of his wife, a black woman who loves him. Reitu, who is from South Africa, helped modify his diet by preparing more of the vegetarian foods she was raised on. She also tries hard to make sure that Chris is getting enough physical activity with her and their young son.

Nearly 3.2 million black Americans over the age of twenty, or 11.4 percent of all black Americans, have diabetes. And over a third of them don't know it. There is a strong link between heart disease, stroke, high blood pressure, and diabetes. Heart attack is the leading cause of death for people living with diabetes. People living with diabetes are two to four times more likely to have heart disease or have a stroke, and 73 percent of all diabetics have some form of high blood pressure.

WHAT IS DIABETES?

Diabetes is a chronic disease in which your body will make very little or no insulin, or is not able to properly use the insulin it makes. Insulin is a hormone that is produced by the pancreas and it helps your body process and use the energy that it gets from sugar. If the body is not making insulin or not using it properly, the body's glucose levels build up over time.

If the man in your life has a family health history of diabetes, is overweight, or is over forty-five, he may be at higher risk for diabetes, and should be screened. When black men have diabetes, they're also much more likely to develop one or more of the serious complications associated with the disease, including kidney failure, blindness, and cardiovascular disease, and even amputation (black Americans are 1.5 to 2.5 times more likely to have a limb amputated than others with diabetes). So the sooner they get a diagnosis, begin regular monitoring and treatment, the more they will be able to work to prevent the very serious complications of diabetes.

There are two types of diabetes.

Type 1 Diabetes

Type 1 diabetes happens when the body's immune system kills off the cells that produce insulin in the pancreas. Once the pancreas no longer produces insulin, sugar builds up in the blood, causing major damage to internal organs. Although anybody can be diagnosed with type 1 diabetes, most are diagnosed during childhood or their teen years. Type 1 diabetes is rarer in blacks.

Type 2 Diabetes

Type 2 diabetes, the more common form of diabetes, accounts for more than 90 percent of all cases. It has almost become an epidemic among both black men and black women, so we need to take special care in understanding this disease and how to manage it. The chances are great that someone in your life either has been affected by type 2 diabetes or will be in the future. Type 2 diabetes is usually diagnosed in adults. But with the high rate of obesity in our children, the medical community is starting to see more adult-onset diabetes in adults and teens.

Black men need to know how to prevent type 2 diabetes and how to control it if they already have it. Both black men and black women must move beyond thinking that just because other members of their family have battled diabetes that they have to get it, too. It isn't necessarily a given. People who have a family history of diabetes also usually have some family lifestyle indicators, such as being overweight or sedentary.

There are things that you can do to prevent it for yourselves, the men in your life, and for your children. People with type 2 diabetes do produce insulin. It's just that the insulin their bodies produce is either not enough to support the body, or their bodies don't recognize that the insulin is there and do not use it. Without insulin, glucose cannot get to the cells in the body. Treating diabetes means regulating blood sugar levels.

If diabetes is not controlled and managed, the high blood sugar levels can cause serious damage to the blood vessels and nerves, and other health complications such as blindness, kidney failure, heart disease, and stroke, as well as the need for amputation of the lower extremities.

WHAT ARE THE SYMPTOMS?

So many men of color are living with pre-diabetes (a fasting blood sugar level of 100 mg/dl, a condition that can lead to type 2 diabetes or diabetes) and don't know it. People may actually live with type 2 diabetes for seven to ten years before it is diagnosed. By the time a man is diagnosed, he may already be experiencing complications. It is important for the women who love him to be aware of the symptoms and warning signs. They can be one or all of these:

- Frequent urination
- Increased thirst and/or hunger
- Unexplained weight loss or gain
- Feeling tired and weak
- Blurred vision
- Dry mouth
- Hard, heavy breathing
- Loss of consciousness
- Slow-healing sores or cuts
- Itchy skin in the groin area
- Numbness or tingling in hands and feet
- Impotence or erectile dysfunction

GETTING SCREENED FOR DIABETES

Diabetes is screened through blood tests at your health care provider's office. The current standards for routine screening for diabetes from organizations such as the American Diabetes Association are that screening begin at age forty-five and occur every three years. However, because blacks are at higher risk, the man in your life should discuss more frequent screenings, that begin earlier, with his physician, if he has any of the risk factors, a family history of diabetes, or is having warning signs of the disease. There are two kinds of tests; one is a random blood sugar test and the other is one that is done while you are fasting. The Fasting Plasma Glucose blood test is the preferred test for diagnosing type 2 diabetes. Table 8.1 shows the different levels and what they mean in terms of his health.

Table 8.1 FASTING PLASMA GLUCOSE TEST	
Plasma Glucose Result (mg/dl)	Diagnosis
99 and below	Normal
100 to 125	Pre-diabetes (impaired fasting glucose)
126 and above	Diabetes*

*Confirmed by repeating the test on a different day.

Research has shown that the Oral Glucose Tolerance Test (OGTT) is more sensitive than the FPG test for diagnosing pre-diabetes, but it is less convenient to administer. The OGTT requires fasting for at least eight hours before the test. A blood test will then measure plasma glucose levels immediately before and two hours after drinking a liquid containing glucose dissolved in water. Table 8.2 illustrates the levels and corresponding diagnosis.

Table 8.2 ORAL GLUCOSE TOLERANCE TEST	
2-Hour Plasma Glucose Result (mg/dl)	**Diagnosis**
139 and below	Normal
140 to 199	Pre-diabetes (impaired glucose tolerance)
200 and above	Diabetes*

*Confirmed by repeating the test on a different day.

HOW CAN I HELP HIM CONTROL IT?

Before we get into the nitty-gritty of how you can help, let us remind you that dealing with diabetes can sometimes feel overwhelming for the person who is living with it. It can be a roller-coaster ride for anyone, especially a newly diagnosed person. Of course we know that people who have support in place do better for longer than people who are out there trying to go it alone. Diabetes management is no exception.

There will probably be days that the man in your life will feel anger about his condition. He may even resent your help and support. Asking for and accepting help is a hard step to take for many men. But it can make a huge difference. Even if he doesn't reach out, you should.

J. Anthony Brown, one of the scream-out-loud, funny personalities on the Tom Joyner radio show, has been dealing with diabetes since 1990. He says that his friends and family members have made a huge difference in his acceptance of his diabetes and in the way he takes care of himself. "I call them my diabetic soldiers. I get five or six calls every morning from different family members," J. Anthony says. "Did you take your medicine? They're like the police."

HELP HIM STOP IT IN ITS TRACKS

First, let us say that even with a family history of diabetes, it can be prevented in many cases. If the man in your life is being monitored regularly by his doctor, he or she can detect that there may be a higher risk for diabetes. He may even be diagnosed with pre-diabetes, which means that there is a high risk for diabetes, but there is an opportunity to change things before your man is actually considered diabetic. Staying on top of diabetes risks is the best preventative action to protect him from the complications that affect black men every day.

Diabetes can result in a mixed bag of emotions for a man living with it and for the women who love and care about him. The National Institutes of Health and the Centers for Disease Control have combined forces for a powerful education program that opens up the dialogue in black communities around diabetes and diabetes management. The training that accompanies a video called *The Debilitator* addresses what goes on in families that face diabetes. This training cites the various stages that a man goes through in dealing with a diabetes diagnosis:

• Denial
• Depression
• Anger
• Bargaining
• Acceptance

TREATING DIABETES

If the man in your life does have diabetes, you can be a great help to him in controlling it, like helping him watch his diet, supporting him in a regular exercise routine, and making sure that he stays at a healthy weight. Many people who are living with type 2 diabetes are able to control it with medication. Some take pills, others regularly test their blood and give themselves insulin through injections. Many diabetics manage their sugar levels with a combination of the two. His doctor will work with him to determine which form of controlling his diabetes is best.

Remind him to keep testing his blood often during the day and keep his blood sugars as near to normal by eating right and taking his medication when needed. People who are living with diabetes really must work closely with their doctors. Help the diabetic man in your life to keep his appointments and go in when he is scheduled for the lab work that your doctor has ordered.

It is important to maintain a healthy diet. A diet that is out of sync can cause huge problems for a diabetic and can raise his blood sugar to dangerous levels. Most of the recommendations for living a heart-healthy diet are the same for diabetics. Experts suggest that a man living with diabetes eat four to five smaller meals a day. They also suggest that patients cut way back on sugar and salt. He should also watch the amount of fat that he eats. Nutritionists and medical experts suggest that no more than 30 percent of the calories he takes in each day come from fat.

Many women who are helping a man in their lives manage his diabetes do so by planning out the meals each day and keeping a strict eye on food quality and portion size. It might even be helpful to set up a consultation or two with a nutritionist who works with diabetes patients or enroll in a diabetes management education program at your local hospital until you get the hang of it.

Take the time to become an expert so that you can help him become an expert, too. Knowing as much as possible about changes to make and things to look out for that may signal the beginning of complications in diabetes self-management goes a long way. Many current resources can help guide you.

One of our goals, as women who are helping men to accept and manage their diabetes, is to work with them to get rid of all their misconceptions about diabetes and necessary treatment. One big myth is that people who use insulin have the "worst kind of diabetes." Insulin is actually the most effective way for a person who has high blood sugar levels to be able to control them quickly.

Kendall Simmons, a member of the 2006 Super–Bowl winning Pittsburgh Steelers, found out that he had diabetes after his rookie year in the NFL. His first symptom was that he started dropping weight suddenly. "I didn't have any energy. I was working hard, doing everything I wanted to, then all of a sudden I couldn't get up and do anything," Kendall says.

His blood glucose levels fluctuated constantly. Kendall says he had all the other symptoms, too, including running to the bathroom every five minutes, being so thirsty that he was drinking everything he could get his hands on, and then after all he drank, still feeling "like I was just eating towels all day."

His wife, Celesta, didn't know what was going on, but she was worried. "He dropped forty-five pounds," she says. It was after he went to the hospital and the medical team ran tests that they found out that his sugar levels were 600. The normal range for a person who does not have diabetes is between 70 and 120.

Celesta says that once they knew what they were dealing with, "Kendall kept doing his job on the gridiron and I would do my job on the grill." She prepares healthy, low-fat meals, and is constantly helping him monitor his sugar levels.

She says she met the most resistance from Kendall when it came to snacks. "He's a snacker," she says. "I still have a struggle with him about it. Sometimes I'd go and check the armrest in his car and find cookies."

Kendall says that sometimes it gets rough because he resists the restraints that diabetes and Celesta have put on him. "Why can't I just be normal and eat what I want to eat?" he says. "She stays on me a lot for what I need to eat and where to watch it."

Like many women, Celesta can just look at her man and know when he is not feeling well. "I say, 'Kendall, go check your sugar. You don't need to eat that. Leave it alone. Why are you drinking that?'" Celesta works hard to provide Kendall the support he needs to manage his diabetes, in a way that he might not be able to do on his own. They work as a team, and the payoff is that Kendall has been able to control the disease, diabetes does not control him.

DIABETES-RELATED CONDITIONS

Foot disease is the most common cause of hospitalization for individuals living with diabetes, and it often results in amputation. But this like many of the other complications of the disease can be avoided with mindful care. The need for amputation comes from poor circulation, nerve damage, or poor healing of foot ulcers or sores in the feet that can all accompany diabetes. If you are helping a man in your life manage diabetes, it is really important to make sure that foot care is a part of the deal. If he has pain in his calves when he walks or changes in his feet—such as thickened nails or fungus infections—he needs to be seen right away.

Remind him to make sure to get the health care provider to check his feet during each visit. The provider should be checking the bottoms of the feet, looking for unusual swelling, asking about blood in the shoes or socks. But even if he or she for some reason doesn't ask, it is crucial that the man in your life (or you) tell the doctor about any unusual symptoms. By reporting symptoms and getting treatment early—at the first sign of trouble—you can help to prevent amputation.

There is good news for those men who will be helped by special shoes that prevent rubbing and ulcers on the foot. If he is eligible, Medicare will pay for 80 percent of the cost of special shoes and inserts that will help to prevent foot or leg amputation.

Diabetic Retinopathy

Diabetes is one of the major reason for loss of vision. Diabetics who have uncontrolled blood sugar levels and high blood pressure are at high risk for blindness. One of twelve people over forty years of age with diabetes will develop diabetic retinopathy, which is caused by damage to the blood vessels in the eye.

Good eye care is important for all men and women, but men with diabetes need a yearly eye exam that includes dilation. In this examination the ophthalmologist dilates the pupils of the eyes to look at the retinal blood vessels for any breakdown, leaks, hemorrhages, or blockages. The best ways to prevent severe diabetic retinopathy are keeping the diabetes under control and monitoring blood sugar levels.

Diabetic Neuropathy

Diabetic neuropathy is nerve damage caused by the disease and its complications. Some of those factors include heredity, diet, and other medical conditions, such as high blood pressure.

Symptoms depend on the type of neuropathy and which nerves are affected. Some people have no symptoms at all. For others, numbness, tingling, or pain in the feet is often the first sign that they are having complications.

The following symptoms may indicate diabetic neuropathy:

- Numbness, tingling, or pain in the toes, feet, legs, hands, arms, and fingers
- Wasting of the muscles of the feet or hands
- Indigestion, nausea, or vomiting
- Diarrhea or constipation
- Dizziness or faintness due to a drop in postural (positional) blood pressure
- Problems with urination
- Erectile dysfunction (impotence)
- Weakness

Kidney Failure

Diabetes is the most common cause of kidney failure, accounting for more than 40 percent of new kidney failure cases. Black men living with diabetes have a higher than average rate of kidney disease or failure. Scientists have not been able to explain these higher rates. The best way to prevent kidney failure is to manage the diabetes and his blood pressure to keep the kidneys from having to work so hard. Think about cutting way back on animal protein, which tends to tax the kidneys.

Medical experts have found that high blood pressure and high levels of blood glucose increase the risk that a person with diabetes will progress to kidney failure. Even when drugs and diet are able to control diabetes, the disease can lead to kidney failure. Most people with diabetes do not develop nephropathy that is severe enough to cause kidney failure. About 17 million people in the United States have diabetes, and over 100,000 people are living with kidney failure as a result of diabetes. Dr. Sandra Gadson, a nephrologist, says that people with diabetes who also have kidney disease undergo either dialysis, which substitutes for some of the filtering functions of the kidneys, or transplantation to receive a healthy donor kidney. Most United States citizens who develop kidney failure are eligible for federally funded health care.

ALCOHOL USE, DIABETES, AND BLACK MEN . . .

There are so many dos and don'ts when it comes to diabetes, but here is one that we must mention specifically—alcohol use. Drinking in moderation is okay if you take proper precautions. The American Diabetes Association reports that alcohol use can be incorporated into an overall diet, if the blood sugar is consistently controlled and monitored.

But we all know someone who has diabetes, or as they call it in our communities, "sugar," who is also a heavy drinker. These men are putting themselves at great risk for many of the complications from diabetes that could end their lives. Trying to deal with diabetes and controlling alcohol can almost be too much. That's why doctors usually recommend to black men who are diabetic that they limit alcohol intake. Make sure the man in your life consults with his health care provider on the recommended and acceptable amounts of alcohol that are right for him.

COMMUNITIES CAN MAKE A DIFFERENCE . . .

Community groups, social organizations, religious groups and their health ministries—any place that people gather—can have a big impact on helping to reduce the risks of chronic illnesses, including diabetes. All over the country, programs are starting up to help people of color become more educated about reducing their risks for diabetes, and providing support to those who have already been diagnosed. If your community does not have programs going on, maybe you can help start one. If they already exist, work to get the men in your life who are at risk, or who have been diagnosed, involved.

If the larger community can have an impact on the health of a person living with diabetes, what could we women do to support our men? If we took the time to learn the dos and don'ts, the ins and outs of living successfully with diabetes, what kind of impact could we make, one house at a time, in keeping our men healthier longer? We can do this together.

TIPS

- Take a diabetes management class together at the hospital or clinic or in one of the community-based programs.
- If you have access to one, consult with a nutritionist who has expertise in diabetes management.
- Remind your man to monitor his blood sugar.
- Help him with a dietary plan for the day. Pack him healthy snacks to take with him.
- Make sure that he has everything he needs to test his blood sugar levels during the day. Many people keep a testing kit at home and one either in their car or at their office so that they are never without this essential tool.
- Help him see the benefits of exercising. Physical ac-

tivity is an important part of a diabetes management plan.
- Make sure he keeps his regularly scheduled doctor appointments. This is where the doctors are able to monitor him for the first stages of any complications, including kidney function or eye problems.

Diabetes

Just because other family members have had diabetes, it does not mean that history has to keep repeating itself. By making lifestyle changes, a man can reduce his risks of being diagnosed with the disease before it starts, turning the tide on diabetes. And even if he is diabetic, by taking extra care, he doesn't have to suffer the debilitating effects of the disease such as blindness, kidney failure, amputation, and death from complications. Losing just 10 percent of his body weight can make a huge difference in preventing, delaying, or managing diabetes.

Here are a few tips:

- Reduce food portion sizes. Use smaller plates. Don't go back for seconds.
- Get rid of the junk and eat higher quality food. Keep meat, fish, and poultry servings to three ounces or the size of a deck of cards.
- Take the salt off the table. Cut back on "hidden" salts that lurk in canned chicken stock, crackers, chips, and other food products.

- Eat smaller desserts or share a single dessert.
- Cut back on fried foods.
- Drink a glass of water ten minutes before eating to take the edge off appetite.
- Learn how to eat fast foods. Go for the healthier food choices, such as salad with dressing on the side.
- Stop eating in front of the television.
- Think about the food. Eat slower. Enjoy every bite. Give the body a chance to realize that it is full.

CHAPTER 9

Cancer

Cancer is the general term for the uncontrolled, abnormal growth of cells within the body. These cells can spread through the bloodstream or lymphatic system. In truth, there are more than 100 different types of diseases that are categorized as cancer. Over 137,000 black Americans were diagnosed with some form of cancer in 2005. Approximately 63,000 black men and black women will lose their battle with the disease each year.

Many cancer deaths are preventable through early detection and aggressive treatment. Fortunately the messages about screening and detection are getting out within our communities now more than ever. Cancer rates are dropping among black men and black women, but the numbers still lag behind the more significant drops among white men and white women.

We are still losing too many of our black men to cancer. Black women have a lot of work to do to get our husbands, fathers, brothers, sons, and friends to take prevention, screening, and treatment seriously. Awareness is key. In this chapter we will help raise your awareness of the top cancer killers of black men in this country— prostate, lung, and colorectal cancers—and ways that you can help the men in your life make steps to prevent or beat these diseases. It can be done. Look around you. There are plenty of survival stories and you will be able to read some of them here. You will also see that the gentle guidance of black women was often at the core of men's survival.

But first, let's explain three key parts of the cancer equation—the oncologist, who is the physician who directs the cancer care, and chemotherapy, and radiation, which are the primary modes of treatment for all forms of cancer.

ONCOLOGISTS

A board certified oncologist is trained to diagnose and treat cancer and goes through rigorous training and examinations to specialize in a specific area of treatment.

There are several kinds of oncologists and many subspecialties of cancer treatment. A *medical oncologist*, who uses medical procedures and chemotherapy treatment, completes specialized training and is certified by the American Board of Internal Medicine. A *radiation oncologist* uses radiation to treat the specific site of the cancer, and is certified by the American Board of Radiology. A *surgical oncologist* works to diagnose a cancer through biopsy and remove it with surgery. Surgical oncologists are certified through the American Board of Surgery. Often a surgical oncologist will remove a tumor and refer the patient to a medical or radiation oncologist for chemotherapy or radiation to kill any cancer cells left.

We recommend using a board certified oncologist. If you want to check the certification of a given oncologist, contact the American Board of Medical Specialties at www.abms.org. They have a list of board certified doctors that you can search by state and specialty.

Choosing the Right Oncologist

Before you start searching for a surgeon or an oncologist, think about the qualities you want your doctor to have. The American Cancer Society offers this list of suggestions, but you may want to add others.

• Your doctor must have experience with your type of cancer. Studies show these doctors have better success treating a condition.
• Your doctor should be part of your health plan and/or accept your health insurance. Otherwise, you need to be prepared to pay for your health care yourself.
• Your doctor should have privileges (is permitted to practice) at a hospital that you find acceptable. Doctors can send patients only to facilities where they have admitting privileges.

• Your doctor must make you feel comfortable. Some people prefer their doctors to have a businesslike manner, while others value a physician who can attend to both their emotional health and their medical needs. Many people whose illnesses require long-term treatment prefer this kind of friendly relationship with their physician.

Get Referrals

One of the best ways to identify a surgeon and/or oncologist is through referrals from people you trust, like your primary care doctor. You might even try to speak with other patients in your community who have been treated for your type of cancer to see who they used.

If you are in a health plan, check their list of doctors, which is usually available online or by calling the member services hotline. Once you've identified doctors that seem like a good fit for you, call their offices and find out whether they are covered by your health plan and are taking new patients. You may also want to find out which hospitals they are affiliated with if that is important to you. It's helpful to ask around about a doctor's reputation, but in the end, trust your gut. You should feel comfortable not only with your doctor's ability to treat your cancer but also with how he or she treats you as a person. If it doesn't feel right, keep looking.

The American Medical Association (AMA), which represents many doctors in the United States, offers a doctor locator service. You can find information about doctors, such as their contact information, medical school, residency training, and specialty area(s). Don't forget to contact the National Medical Association, the association that represents black physicians, including oncologists.

Another source of information is the American Society of Clinical Oncology. This is an international medical society representing cancer specialists involved in clinical research and patient care. They provide an oncologist directory, which is a database of ASCO members.

The next step is to schedule appointments with a few doctors. The most important question to ask them is whether they have experience treating the type of cancer that the man in your life has. If you are meeting with surgeons, find out how often they perform the type of surgery you need, how many of these surgeries they have performed before, and what their success rate is.

In addition to finding out your doctor's medical qualifications, take note of how comfortable you are with him or her. One way to gauge this is to answer the following questions after your appointment:

• Did the doctor give you a chance to ask questions?
• Did you feel like the doctor was listening to you?
• Did the doctor seem comfortable answering your questions?
• Did the doctor talk to you in a way that you could understand?
• Did you feel like the doctor respected you?
• Did the doctor ask your preferences about different kinds of treatments?

• Did you feel like the doctor spent enough time with you?

Trust yourselves when deciding whether this doctor is right for him. Keep in mind, though, that relationships take time to develop and you may need more than one visit before you and your doctor really get to know each other.

Is the Oncologist Board Certified?

Oncologists who are board certified have been trained in special treatment areas. They have taken and passed certification examinations given by doctors in their field. To keep their certification, doctors must continue their education.

Not all oncologists who are specialists are board certified. Doctors do not need to be board certified to be excellent caregivers. Still, more than 85 percent of doctors are board certified in at least one specialty.

To find out if an oncologist that you are considering is board certified, contact the American Board of Medical Specialties (ABMS) (www.abms.org). The ABMS has a list of board certified doctors who subscribe to the ABMS service. You can search for all doctors in a certain specialty by state. Or you can type in the name of the doctor to learn about his specialty. Information on doctors who have additional training and certification may also be available at your public library. Ask for the *Official ABMS Directory of Board Certified Medical Specialists*, or ask your librarian to help you.

If you are still unsure, you can find out who are the leading authorities in the field. A visit to a medical library may be useful. Consider doing research on the Internet as well. Look for doctors who have written about the cancer affecting your life and whose work is most often quoted. If your doctor has done research and had it published, you may ask to see copies of those articles. By doing so, you will learn more about their approach to cancer treatment.

With What Hospitals Is the Oncologist Affiliated?

Where you will receive inpatient cancer care is determined by where your doctor practices. Find out where you would go for surgery or other care. Check with your health insurance company to see which doctors and hospitals your insurance plan covers.

Is the Oncologist Affiliated with a Medical School?

Teaching affiliation with a respected medical school may suggest a doctor that is a leader in his or her field. Doctors who teach and who also practice medicine often are in contact with medical experts from around the country. They may know more about the latest treatments.

Other Questions to Ask

• Are you or your practice involved in clinical trials (medical studies) of new treatments?
• What are your office hours?
• How can the doctor be contacted after hours?
• Who will see me when the doctor is on vacation?
• Who else will be on my health care team?

You might also contact the nearest cancer centers and ask for doctors who are specialists in your type of cancer. Consider asking family, friends, nurses, and other doctors in your community. Most hospitals also have a doctor referral service. Or call medical schools or medical societies in your area. Once you have come up with some names, you might begin getting the answers to some of the same questions you asked before, for example, board certification and experience.

CHEMOTHERAPY

Chemotherapy is a popular treatment option that uses strong chemicals or drugs to prevent the reproduction of cancer cells and stop their growth. Chemotherapy can be used in conjunction with radiation therapy and surgery. These drugs are often given in different combinations to more effectively attack the cancer. The size of a tumor, stage of the disease, and overall health of the patient will be considered by a patient's oncologist when determining the most effective treatment plan.

Chemotherapy drugs may be given intravenously or

taken orally in tablet, capsule, or liquid form. As chemotherapy drugs circulate through the entire body by way of the bloodstream, they may reach cancer cells missed by surgery or radiation treatment.

The amount of chemotherapy a patient receives depends on the type of cancer, the drugs, and his overall response to treatment. Chemotherapy may be given daily, weekly, or monthly, and can continue for months or even years. Some drugs may be given in cycles—with rest periods in between treatments—to allow the body to recover and produce new, healthy cells.

Side effects vary depending on the type of chemotherapy and how the patient responds. A medical oncologist will explain the most common side effects of a particular treatment. Chemotherapy side effects may be extremely uncomfortable, but most symptoms are temporary and gradually disappear after the treatment ends. During therapy, patients should discuss with the members of their treatment team any side effects they experience. There are medicines available to help manage the discomforts, such as Procrit.

Some common side effects associated with chemotherapy include:

• *Nausea and vomiting*. Chemotherapy may cause nausea and vomiting, which the doctor can help prevent or lessen by prescribing a variety of treatments. Eating is very important to provide strength to help the patient feel better. To lessen symptoms, eat and drink slowly and avoid eating fried or fatty foods. A patient might try eating many small meals as opposed to big meals each day. After eating, it is important to not lie down flat for at least two hours, as this may worsen symptoms.

- *Hair loss.* Hair loss can occur on all parts of the body. Sometimes hair falls out completely, while other times the hair grows thinner. In most cases, hair grows back after the treatment is completed, but may be a different texture and/or thickness.
- *Fatigue.* Chemotherapy affects the bone marrow and the body's ability to produce red blood cells, which may temporarily cause a condition called anemia. Anemia often makes patients feel weak and tired. It is important to get more sleep at night and rest during the day to lessen fatigue. Eating foods rich in iron and regular exercise have also been shown to help combat fatigue.
- *Infections.* The effect of chemotherapy on bone marrow may also lower the amount of white blood cells, which help fight infection. To prevent infection, patients should avoid exposure to people who have a cold, flu, or any other contagious diseases. Frequent hand washing can also help minimize infection.
- *Bleeding.* Chemotherapy can affect other blood cells called platelets, which may lead to easier bruising or bleeding. If bleeding occurs, report it to the treatment team immediately.

RADIATION THERAPY

Radiation therapy is an effective treatment for many kinds of cancer. It involves the use of high-energy X-rays (much stronger than the X-rays used to image teeth or bones) to kill cancer cells or prevent them from growing.

Specialized doctors, called radiation oncologists or radiation therapists, use advanced equipment to target the X-rays directly at tumors or anywhere cancer is present. The treatment is meant to destroy the cancer cells with minimal radiation exposure to healthy cells. Although special shields help protect parts of the body not requiring treatment, some healthy cells will be damaged by the X-rays.

Radiation treatment is often spaced over a number of weeks or months, allowing the healthy cells that may be affected to have time to rejuvenate. The number of treatments a patient receives depends on the type and extent of the tumor, as well as the radiation dosage and how the patient's tolerance is affected by the treatment.

Side Effects of Radiation

Depending on the patient's therapy program, side effects may vary. Some may be severe, but often disappear over a period of time once the therapy is now completed. Side effects should be described to the doctor immediately so that he or she can help minimize them as best as possible through medicines or a change in diet.

Some common side effects associated with radiation therapy include:

• *Fatigue.* Fatigue is the most common side effect associated with radiation therapy. A patient undergoing radiation should rest as much as possible at night and limit their activities during the day.

- *Eating problems.* While nausea may occur with radiation therapy, it is important to eat so that the body has enough nutrients to repair damaged cells. Instead of big meals, patients should try eating many small meals throughout the day. The treatment team can help determine if a special diet is needed (no spicy or fatty foods) and may suggest how to maintain a healthy weight. Medicine to prevent nausea can also be prescribed.
- *Hair loss.* Loss of hair may occur in the direct path of the radiation.
- *Skin reaction.* The skin in the treatment area may become dry, irritated, and sensitive, and should be treated gently. Patients should bathe carefully, using only warm water and mild soap, and avoid all cosmetics, lotions, and deodorants. The affected area should be kept out of direct sunlight for at least one year after treatment.

LUNG CANCER

Linda Weatherspoon Haithcox still talks about losing her father to lung cancer as if it happened yesterday. Linda says her father had actually been diagnosed in the 1950s, but the medical experts did not insist on treatment at the time. She also adds that her father never stopped smoking. He eventually developed a terrible cough and the family urged and cajoled him into going to the doctor. "He didn't want to go. He didn't want to know," she says. "But he got sicker and sicker."

By the time he was officially diagnosed, he was in the end stages of the disease. "I will always wonder what would have happened if he had stopped smoking—for us," she says.

Black men are at least 50 percent more likely to develop lung cancer than white males and are 36 percent more likely to die from the disease, according to the American Lung Association. Sometimes environmental hazards cause lung cancer, such as asbestos, or chemicals used in factories and plants, but the real deal is that 90 percent of lung cancers are caused by smoking. Which means that 90 percent of all lung cancer diagnoses and deaths among our black men is preventable.

At over 163,000 deaths each year, lung cancer kills more people in the United States than breast, prostate, and colorectal cancers combined. A recent study suggests that two-thirds of all cancer deaths could be eliminated if black men would give up tobacco. It's not just lung cancer. A smoker has a higher risk of throat, mouth, and bladder cancer.

If we could just get black men to stop smoking, or for that matter to never start, we could save the lives of thousands of people a year. We also know that smoking contributes to high blood pressure, heart disease, asthma, and stroke, all things that our black men suffer from at disproportionately high rates.

Are we trying to scare you? Yes. Ladies, this is an area where we have to really roll up our sleeves and be advocates for and to our men about their health.

Screening and Detection

The five-year survival rate for a man with lung cancer, who is diagnosed before it has spread to other parts of the body, is 50 percent. Unfortunately only 15 percent of lung cancers are found in their early stages. The good news is that when lung cancer is caught in its earliest stages, and early surgery can be preformed, the survival rates go up to 85 percent. There are several procedures that can be done to screen for and detect lung cancer.

Your man's health care provider will do a physical examination, looking for swollen lymph nodes in the neck and collarbone area, and ask key questions about his overall health. This would be followed up by a chest exam where the provider listens to the lungs through a stethoscope, in order to hear any abnormal breathing patterns.

The physician may also ask him to cough up some phlegm, to examine under a microscope, looking for abnormal or cancerous cells. He may also be given a chest X-ray, which is an imaging test in order to see the lungs and identify any suspicious growths.

Or he may be given a more sensitive, detailed CT scan, or a magnetic resonance imaging (MRI) test, which gives a two-dimensional image of the lungs. These tests may pick up some abnormal growths that a traditional X-ray may not be able to. He may also be given a bronchoscopy, where the physician can actually view the lungs through a hollow tube that goes through the nose and throat, into the main airways of the lungs.

If the physician has additional reason for concern, he will order a lung biopsy, which is a surgical procedure to remove some lung tissue, and look at it under a microscope.

In a diagnosis of limited small cell lung cancer, the tumor is found in one lung and in nearby lymph nodes. In the case of a diagnosis of extensive small cell lung cancer, the tumor has already spread to the other lung and other organs of the body.

In non–small cell cancers, there are five stages:

- *Stage I a/b.* The tumor, no matter what its size, is contained in only the lung.
- *Stage II a/b.* The tumor has spread to the closest lymph nodes or the other lung, or even the neck and is graded according to its size and whether or not it has spread to the chest wall or outer covering of the lung.
- *Stage III.* The tumor has spread to the lymph nodes in the trachea, into the chest wall, and in the diaphragm.
- *Stage III b.* Can mean there is more than one tumor or that it has grown into another major organ.
- *Stage IV.* The tumor has spread beyond the chest.

Treatment

Lung cancer is usually treated with surgery, chemotherapy, and/or several weeks of radiation, depending on the individual patient.

Surgery can offer the greatest chance for a cure for many types of lung cancer, especially if the cancer has not yet spread or metastasized to other parts of the body. Surgery cannot be used as a cure, but can treat complications seen in advanced disease. Most patients will undergo some type of surgery throughout the course of their diagnosis and treatment.

There are three general types of surgery for lung cancer. First, curative surgery which can be used to remove the cancerous tumor, and perhaps a part of or the entire lung. Second, debulking surgery is used when the entire tumor is too big to remove. The surgeons will remove part of the tumor and the other portion will then be treated with chemotherapy or radiation to shrink it. Finally, sometimes surgeons will perform surgery on a tumor that is causing pain or disability.

But It's Tough to Stop . . .

Most smokers are aware of the deadly risks, and in fact have tried to quit at least once in their lives. It usually takes several tries. We must support them again and again and again as they try to kick this nasty and deadly habit. Saying no and being able to follow through is a hard thing to do.

The National Cancer Institute says that it can be harder to break a nicotine/cigarette habit than it is to shake heroin or cocaine. It may take up to four attempts before a person can kick the habit.

Smoking is an addiction on two levels. We now know that some of the chemicals in cigarettes are there because they reinforce the dependence and addiction. A man has a cigarette to help relax and unwind after a hard day. He reaches for a cigarette after a meal and as a stress reliever. If he is reaching for anything that much, simply put, he is probably addicted to it. Although it is socially more acceptable than a heroin or crack addiction, smoking is equally deadly. Tobacco use kills more black people than other illegal drug addictions. Think about that for a minute.

How Do I Help Him Stop?

Here is the important thing that we really have to remember. In many of the other areas we can help our men, we can make subtle changes that they don't even notice to get them jump-started. There are many effective products on the market that can help reduce the urge to smoke, including gum, patches, inhalers, and tablets. These products give the body just enough nicotine to quench the craving without giving it the damaging tar and carbon monoxide buildup that contributes to lung cancer.

But his smoking habit is all about him. He has to genuinely want to and be ready to stop smoking. You can help him develop a plan; you can buy him the nicotine patches that are available to help him wean himself off the cigarettes. But until he's ready, you are wasting your time.

But there is something powerful that you can do (in addition to getting the patches and the nicotine gum ready). Give him real and urgent reasons to stop. Tell him from your heart how scared you and your family are for him. Explain to him what losing him to lung cancer or emphysema would do to you. Just saying it won't be enough for him to stop, but it will give him a really strong motivation, stronger than yelling at him about making your car smell like smoke. (Been there, done that!)

Once he does decide to try to quit, be a support for him. He has taken on one of the toughest behavior modification tasks there is when he agrees to give up the smokes. But he will need support. Truth be told, he may be hard to live with in those first thirty days. People who have stopped have told us that the first week or two are just awful. He may also have some false starts, but we can help him pick himself up and start over.

And this is obvious, but we will say it anyway. If you are a smoker, even if you smoke one just every now and then, you have to stop, too—especially if you want him to quit.

Another motivator for parents is their children. Our children watch our example. They learn by modeling our behaviors. Children who smoke at a young age have often gotten it from their parents. And studies show that bad habits that are picked up young, like smoking and uncontrolled alcohol use, are hard habits to kick later. Plus, just think of the lung damage a lifetime of smoking could do to your child.

Finally, it is helpful to remind him of the dangers of secondhand smoke. Being around smoke and smokers can have devastating effects for others. The CDC says that thousands of people die of secondhand smoke–related causes each year, including lung cancer. Pediatricians suggest that children who have asthma are more likely to have severe asthma attacks if they are around cigarette smoke.

Be an Advocate

The tobacco companies aren't making it any easier for us. As the rates of tobacco use among whites are shrinking, the tobacco industry is dropping big bucks in communities of color to get our young men and women to light up. They have to keep seeking out new markets as old ones shut down. They see the vulnerable black and Hispanic communities as easy targets. We need to say no to ads that promote smoking in our communities much in the way that middle-income white women joined forces with policymakers to create very effective anti-smoking movements and smoke-free zones in their communities. The tobacco companies have often been compared to Goliath, but we black women can become the Davids who run that giant out of our communities for the sake of our families.

Tips for Helping Him Stop

• Have a plan. Maybe the plan is through his doctor. Maybe you research a plan on the Internet or through the American Cancer Society, or Lung Association. Your local health department or hospital may also have a free or low-cost plan that he can follow. Or he may decide that the best plan for him is to go cold-turkey. It is easier to have a plan than to try to stop without one.
• Create smoke-free zones. Ban smoking from the house and the car.
• Keep healthy snacks around to help him satisfy the urge to put something in his mouth.

- Send him walking. Walking is a great tool for people who are trying to stop smoking. It helps them relax, keeps their minds off the cigarettes, and helps prevent the weight gain that some smokers experience.
- Be nice. He may be extremely cranky during this time. It may be up to you to be overly gracious and kind while he makes this change for himself and for you.
- Show him the cost savings. A man who shakes a $4-a-day cigarette habit will save $1,460 a year. Over fifteen years, he has not only continued to reduce his risk for cancer and heart disease, but he has pocketed $21,900 that he would have spent on tobacco products.

PROSTATE CANCER

Reverend Charles Johnson, one of the driving forces behind the Indiana Black Expo organization and the Circle City Classic football game, is a real profile in courage for black men. His poignant and thoughtful book, *That Black Men Might Live*, chronicles his battle with prostate cancer, a battle that in the end claimed his life. In writing the book, he took the time to send a message loud and clear to black men, and to us the women who care for them, that we must take good care of each other. His sister, Kathy Jordan, who is a vice president with the Indiana Pacers basketball organization, says that Charles ignored the warnings that his body was sending him.

"He had these struggles with his weight for so long," Kathy says of her brother, whose weight at its highest had inched up to over 400 pounds. He spent so much time worrying about his weight and a family history of high blood pressure that he ignored other warning signals that his body was giving him about another real threat to his health—prostate cancer. Even though he had a family history of cancer, Kathy says he never really saw it as a personal threat to his life.

"He'd hide his symptoms from us," Kathy says. "He'd diagnose himself, even though he was not a doctor. He'd call his friends who were doctors and say 'I think I have a cold' and get antibiotics," she says.

Kathy says she will never forget the day that she and her mother went with Charles to his follow-up visit with his doctor after his cancer screening tests. The doctor told him not only that he had prostate cancer, but it was in its most advanced stages. The cancer had already spread to his ribs and lymph nodes.

Charles did what many of our black men do. They avoid seeking out care. They also load the deck with miscues and misinformation. Instead of sharing the symptoms with their doctors, they interpret the symptoms even before they walk through the door. "I just have a little cold. I just have a little flu. I just have . . ."

Once Charles and his family got the diagnosis, Kathy says that she hunkered down and did a lot of research. She did her homework so that she could help her brother talk to the doctors and know more about treatment options for prostate cancer. Even with the knowledge she gained, she still wishes that she had been more assertive on her brother's behalf. "The doctors recommended a type of hormonal treatment that is often used in prostate cancer treatment, but I always questioned why they weren't more aggressive. Why didn't they start out with chemotherapy?" Kathy asks.

She says that one of her regrets is following Charles's lead when it came to treatment. "He just wasn't being aggressive, and I didn't want to upset him." Then once she saw that he wasn't getting any better she took stronger action. "I started questioning him about the choices he was making in his health care. If there was a treatment that I thought he ought to be on and if he said no, I'd make him tell me how he came up with that choice." She felt it was important to engage him in making what she calls informed choices about his care.

For every story of what could have been there is a positive story about a man who is beating the odds—with the help of the women who love him. Lonnie Johnson is one of those men. Even though he had worked in public health for many years, and had always been a community advocate for black men's health, he says that in 1994 it was his wife Glen who saved his life.

Although Glen is a physician, it wasn't her medical background that made her insist that Lonnie go for prostate cancer screening. It was because she loves him. He had been putting off getting a routine physical for a while. "But she kept at me until I went to the doctor, and sure enough, I had prostate cancer. I know she saved my life," says Lonnie, who is now considered a long-term survivor.

What Is Prostate Cancer?

The prostate is a sex gland. When it is normal, it is about the size of a walnut. It is located between the bladder and the penis and in front of the rectum. The urethra, the tube that carries urine from the bladder and out of the body through the penis, passes through the center of the prostate. Think of the prostate as the gateway for a man's reproductive and urinary systems.

Prostate cancer is a series of small cancerous tumors that form in the cells of the prostate gland. As long as the cells are contained in the prostate and have not spread to other organs, the cure rate with treatment is at 90 percent. If the cancer spreads to the lymph nodes it becomes more difficult to treat. Without treatment, experts estimate that it takes approximately fifteen to seventeen years to cause death.

Prostate cancer is the most common form of cancer for men in the United States. In fact, more men contract prostate cancer than women develop breast cancer. Black men have the highest rates of prostate cancer of any men in the world, and sadly due to late diagnosis and treatment they die from the disease at a rate that is double their white counterparts. Scientists are not quite sure why our men have a higher rate of prostate cancer than other men, but many feel sure that the death rates could be greatly improved by early screenings and aggressive treatment.

What Puts Black Men at Risk?

Through medical experts can't say for sure what puts our men at higher risk, there are several factors that can contribute. The single biggest factor for all men is age. The older a man is, the more his risk factors go up. It's rare for a man to develop prostate cancer if he is under age fifty. And 80 percent of all prostate cancers are diagnosed in men over sixty-five, with numbers that seem to spike in men over age seventy. But black men have a higher incidence of developing prostate cancer in their fifties. So their screenings should begin at age forty, particularly if there is a family health history of prostate cancer (having two first-generation relatives who have had prostate cancer increases a man's risk) or any symptoms that could be linked to the disease.

Diets high in fat have been linked to prostate cancer. So if we want to help men avoid prostate cancer, like other cancers and chronic diseases, help them reduce the fatty, fried foods they eat. Add more fruit and vegetables to their diet. Foods that are high in fiber or rich in antioxidants like lycopene found in raw or cooked tomatoes can help. Leafy green vegetables like cabbage, broccoli, and sprouts are good additions to a cancer prevention diet, too.

Nutritionists and medical researchers seem to think that by adding soy products that contain isoflavones, like soy milk and soy nuts, to the diet, a man may be able to keep his testosterone levels under control and reduce the risk of cancer. Because prostate cancer feeds off testosterone, isoflavones may reduce the risk and progression of the disease. The goal is to gradually build your level of resistance.

Symptoms

Prostate cancer in its early stages may not carry any warning signs. It tends to be a slow growing cancer that takes years or decades before it causes severe problems, such as painful urination, incontinence, or blood in the urine, that might cause a man to seek out medical attention. But even when it does, our men tend not to share such private information. So needless to say, with men like Charles, many of those warning signs are ignored or shaken off as symptoms of another problem. If he does complain about any of these symptoms, you definitely want to convince him to see his doctor and get screened right away.

Following is a list of prostate cancer symptoms:

- Dull pain in the lower pelvic area
- Urgency of urination
- Difficulty starting urination
- Pain during urination
- Weak urine flow and dribbling
- Intermittent urine flow
- A sensation that the bladder isn't empty immediately after urination
- Frequent urination at night
- Blood in the urine
- Painful ejaculation during sex
- General pain in the lower back, hips, or upper thighs

- Loss of appetite and weight in combination with the other symptoms
- Persistent bone pain

Screening

There are two ways that health care providers can detect prostate cancer. The most common is the digital rectal examination (DRE), where the provider inserts a gloved finger into the rectum of the patient to feel for abnormalities.

The other common screening method is the prostate-specific antigen test, which is a blood test that measures the prostate specific antigen (PSA) enzyme. All men have prostate-specific proteins in their blood, but a healthy man who does not have prostate cancer usually has relatively low levels of the PSA enzyme. The higher the level of PSA the more likely it is that the man has prostate cancer. An elevated PSA does not always signal cancer, however. Some medications and herbal supplements can alter test results. So make sure he tells his health care provider of any medicines, both prescription and over-the-counter, that he may be on before taking a PSA test.

Neither test is a foolproof diagnosis by itself. And the PSA test has been linked with false positive results. But experts have seen strong evidence that the PSA screenings are the best tools we currently have in detecting prostate cancer in its early stages. To confirm the presence of cancer, a health care provider will probably recommend a consultation with a surgeon and having a biopsy of the prostate.

Table 9.1
UNDERSTANDING PSA LEVELS

These numbers represent what doctors consider normal PSA levels in men where no prostate cancer exists. Higher levels on a test may be evidence of prostate cancer and require further tests, often including a biopsy. It is a good idea to keep a personal record of PSA levels over time. Some medications can elevate these levels.

Age	Normal PSA Range
40 and younger	0 to 2.0 ng/mL
45	0 to 2.4 ng/mL
50	0 to 2.8 ng/mL
55	0 to 3.3 ng/mL
60	0 to 3.8 ng/mL
65	0 to 4.5 ng/mL
70	0 to 5.3 ng/mL
75	0 to 6.2 ng/mL
80 and older	0 to 7.2 ng/mL

But the information on prostate cancer screening is mixed and confusing for patients. The Centers for Disease Control walk a fine line when making their recommendations. They promote informed decision making, which they say occurs when a man understands the seriousness of prostate cancer; understands the risks, benefits, and alternatives to screening; participates in decision making to the level he wishes; and makes a decision about screening that is consistent with his preferences. However they do not specifically recommend routine screening for prostate cancer because they say there is no scientific consensus on whether screening and treatment of early stage prostate cancer reduces mortality.

But if you ask black men like Lonnie Johnson, they will say that screening saves lives. Family medicine physicians like Dr. Margaret Aguwa have routinely encouraged their patients, especially their black patients who are over forty, to have a prostate exam every year as a part of their routine physical. So until we get better information, ladies, we need to keep gently guiding our men to screening.

What If He Does Get a Prostate Cancer Diagnosis?

Many notable black men have gotten a prostate cancer diagnosis, but thanks to aggressive treatment and support from their families and friends, have continued to lead rich lives. The Honorable Minister Louis Farrakhan, Harry Belafonte, Nelson Mandela, Colin

Powell, Sidney Poitier, Bishop Desmond Tutu, and former U.N. ambassador and former mayor of Atlanta Andrew Young are all living witnesses to the power of early diagnosis and treatment. Dr. Louis Sullivan, former head of the United States Health and Human Services and outspoken advocate for bridging the gaps in health disparities between people of color and their white counterparts, is also a prostate cancer survivor. Famed pediatric neurosurgeon Dr. Benjamin Carson, who survived prostate cancer surgery, says prostate cancer doesn't have to kill anyone. "The diseases of the prostate gland are eminently treatable if detected early and treated aggressively and appropriately," he says. "There is no reason that a person diagnosed with these diseases cannot live a long, productive, and highly enjoyable life."

In fact, thanks to aggressive screening programs, the light is shining brightly on black men with prostate cancer. With an early diagnosis and treatment, prostate cancer now has a 97 percent cure rate, compared to a 67 percent rate twenty years ago. Together we can help to make sure that more of our wonderful black men are in that 97 percent by helping them catch it early.

Treatment

Ask any wife, sister, or mother of a black man who has had a prostate cancer diagnosis. Just because she may have gotten him to the doctor for screening and diagnosis, does not mean that her work is done. We clearly have a role, like the one Kathy assumed for her brother

Charles, of helping him gather the necessary treatment option information and helping him sort it out to make the best possible choice for him.

As a part of your job as a key member of his support system in this journey, your most important role might just be being his health advocate. Data from University of Michigan and the National Cancer Institute suggest that our fathers, husbands, brothers, sons, and friends are less likely to seek treatment after they receive a diagnosis. In fact, a black man with an early stage cancer is 36 percent less likely to seek treatment than a white man with the same diagnosis. There are many reasons, including issues of health insurance coverage and ability to pay. But another reason that cannot be overlooked is his poor follow-through on the next stages of treatment.

Prostate Cancer Treatment Options

Treatment options vary based on the stage of the tumor. In the early stages, surgical removal of the prostate and radiation may be used to eradicate the tumor. Prostate cancer that has been unsuccessfully treated by hormonal manipulation or has spread to other parts of the body may be treated successfully by chemotherapy. Lonnie says that his diagnosis and reviewing the options for treatment with his wife and his health care provider were frustrating. "We talked to four different urologists," Lonnie says. "Three recommended surgery and one recommended radiology." He opted for surgery.

Surgery

Doctors usually only recommend surgery after thorough evaluation and discussion of treatment options. If this is what your doctor recommends, press the doctor to tell you the benefits of surgery, as well as its potential risks and the side effects.

Removal of the prostate gland (radical prostatectomy) is often recommended for treatment of early stage prostate cancers that have not spread to other parts of the body. One woman we interviewed says that she and her husband were still angry because the doctors never really told them what to expect after the surgery. "He had a terrible time adjusting at first, and it did affect our lives," she says. Some of the side effects of surgery, like the ones her husband experienced at first, are impotence and temporary urinary incontinence. But some of the newer, more specific surgical procedures may be better because they may reduce the risk of these complications.

Terry Mason, MD, a nationally recognized urologist, says that this kind of surgery should be performed by a urologist with extensive experience doing this specific procedure.

Radiation Therapy

Radiation therapy is one option that doctors use to treat prostate cancer. There is still a lot of debate among doctors on the benefits of radiation versus surgery to treat prostate cancer. Some patients of radiation therapy have a loss of appetite, fatigue, skin reactions such as redness and irritation, rectal burning or injury, diarrhea, cystitis, and blood in the urine. A person who opts to have external beam radiation therapy can expect it to be performed five days a week for six to eight weeks.

Another radiation option is implanting small pellets of radioactive iodine, gold, or iridium directly into the prostate tissue through a small surgical incision. The advantage of this radiation therapy is that the radiation is more specific because it is directed at the prostate with less damage to the surrounding tissues.

Radiation Seeds

Many doctors have seen great results with their patients who are given radioactive seeds implanted right into the prostate. The tiny seeds work locally to impact the cancerous prostate cells.

Hormonal Therapy

Hormone therapy, either through surgical removal of the testes or through medications, works to lower testosterone levels. Because prostate tumors need testosterone to grow, reducing the testosterone level is often very effective in preventing further growth and spread of the cancer. The drugs must be given by injection, usually every three months. Possible side effects include nausea and vomiting, hot flashes, anemia, lethargy, osteoporosis, reduced sexual desire, and erectile dysfunction or impotence.

Other medications used for hormonal therapy include androgen-blocking agents, which prevent testosterone from attaching to prostate cells. Possible side effects include erectile dysfunction, loss of sexual desire, liver problems, diarrhea, and enlarged breasts.

Chemotherapy

Doctors also use chemotherapy to treat advanced prostate cancers that have not been treated successfully through radiation, seed implantation, or hormonal treatments and manipulation.

Lifestyle Changes

Surgery, radiation therapy, and hormonal manipulation all have the potential to disrupt sexual desire or performance on either a temporary or permanent basis. Couples and individuals need to have an open and honest conversation about their concerns with their doctor. The fear of loss of sexual desire or ability to perform sexually is one of men's biggest concerns about going through with treatment. Dr. Mason says that there are several options available for men who have "issues" after prostate cancer treatment.

Monitoring

Just like other cancers, the man in your life will be monitored on the status of the disease, no matter what option he chooses. He can expect to come in every three months to a year for a PSA blood test. The doctors will also want to do regular bone scans and CT scans to make sure the cancer has not spread to other parts of the body, and will want to give him a blood test to make sure that he is not suffering from anemia.

If he is undergoing or has been through treatment, you could be a big help to him in looking out for other signs and symptoms that may mean the prostate cancer is progressing, such as being extremely tired, losing weight, increased pain, changed bowel and bladder function, and depression.

Aside from Working Through Treatment with Him, What Can You Do?

- Help him to keep a positive attitude. As scary as a cancer diagnosis may be, reinforce for him that there are lots of living, breathing examples that there is a wonderful life on the other side of prostate cancer.
- Join him in getting exercise and staying physically active. We know that exercise helps fight depression and can help him channel his anger and stress at this time.
- Link him into a strong support system. There may be a group of black men at your church or in his circle of friends who have been through the same thing and are willing to share what they have learned and how they cope with some of the side effects of treatment.
- Encourage him to talk about his feelings and be prepared to listen without judgment. Cancer is too heavy a load to carry alone.
- If you are helping your husband or significant other,

keep the doors to intimate contact open. Prostate cancer is not a death sentence for sex and intimacy. Help him ease his mental pressure to perform. As we know, there are many ways to express our affection for each other. He may experience some initial impotence or erectile dysfunction, but together you can work through this with the help of your health care provider.

COLORECTAL CANCER

Erin Stennis never intended to be a health advocate, or a cancer expert for the African American community. She also never intended to be a young widow raising two children alone.

In November 2001, her husband of fourteen years, Michael Stennis, former college football star and Los Angeles businessman, got a phone call that turned their lives upside down. Michael had had a colonoscopy a few days earlier. The doctor revealed that he had stage IV colon cancer. It had already spread to his liver and lungs. That's when Erin did what every woman who loves her man does. She joined him in the fight of his life.

Even though the odds were against Michael, the couple was determined not only to beat the cancer and get on with their lives, but to use this challenge as an opportunity to reach out to other people of color to talk about colon cancer and how to prevent it. "Our faith was strong, and we felt that we had been chosen to help others," Erin says.

Michael underwent complicated surgery to remove as many of the cancerous tumors in his colon as possible. It was a difficult surgery, and the doctors found more extensive damage than they had anticipated, including some tumors that were too large to remove at that time. After surgery, Michael underwent a year of chemotherapy to shrink the tumors in his liver and lungs. Erin says that those were rough times for everyone. The chemotherapy left Michael weak and worn out many days. "Michael was a man who was an athlete, he was used to making his body work. But during the treatment, he had to learn to give in to what was going on. He had to learn how to rest and let the treatment do its work," Erin says.

Although she says there were many days that he was in pain, and some days that he couldn't even get out of bed because of treatment or the medications used to keep him out of pain, Erin smiles when she thinks of the good days—days between chemo treatments when he felt driven to do something. It was during those days that they worked together to establish and fund a colorectal cancer education campaign in the black community in the Los Angeles area that they called home. "We wanted to make sure what happened to us out of ignorance and lack of information didn't happen to others," says Erin.

"When we started on this journey, neither of us knew that blacks are at increased risk for colon cancer," Erin explains. "Michael was forty-three. We thought he would get tested at age fifty," Erin says. She didn't know that her husband was keeping a deadly secret from her. He had been having symptoms he ignored for about a year before he had the colonoscopy—pain, blood in the stool, which he assumed was related to years of hemorrhoids.

"The truth is, a doctor had recommended that Michael have a colonoscopy during the time when he first had symptoms before, but being a very macho man, he did not want anything invasive. So he didn't get the test, and he didn't tell me that the doctor had suggested it," she says, feeling sure that an earlier intervention could have changed the outcome. The situation was complicated by the fact that there was a history of colon cancer in Michael's family that no one ever talked about—until after he had surgery to remove the colon tumor.

"Michael just couldn't imagine—as many men and women, but especially men, can't—that type of procedure taking place. Of course I wondered why he was going to the doctor so often, not knowing that the doctors suspected that there might be something wrong. When I finally asked him about it, he told me they were going to treat him for hemorrhoids, and that was the end of that." Then, Erin says, Michael's pain became more severe over the following year. "I walked into our bedroom one morning and found him hunched over in the closet in excruciating pain."

Erin says she'll never forget that evening in November, after the results of the colonoscopy were in, and they got that call that led to months of surgery, hospitals, and treatment. "The doctor told us that the cancer was very advanced, and we would be fighting an uphill battle if we were going to beat this. We knew that it didn't look good. He didn't say terminal at that point, but he didn't give us the optimism we would have hoped for," she said.

"Michael sat in his chair and it was just like a cloud came over him. I think my husband stayed in that place for maybe about a week," Erin says. Then she knew she had to kick into high gear and get him in that same mind-set. "I said, 'Okay, let's get information. Let's find out everything we can about this.' And that's what we did. We armed ourselves with information and started fighting."

Where many couples would have decided to retreat, Michael and Erin made a conscious decision to fight this cancer for themselves and for other black men. Erin says that they both spoke at LA area community centers, chambers of commerce, and health fairs, as well as to friends and family—anywhere or any time that Michael's health would permit him to get out and tell his story. "He spread the word as long as his health would allow. He actually went into the pulpit at churches and told our story," she says.

The power of seeing an otherwise visually healthy, strong, and successful man in the throes of a devastating illness was an eye opener for other black men. "People told me, 'You know what? This could be me. So I need to find out more. I need to get screened,'" Erin remembers.

There were times when Michael would rally and experience surges of energy that gave them both hope that the aggressive treatment was working. "It was a roller coaster. Some days we would get bad news—the cancer was spreading, then we would get some little ray of hope that the cancer was shrinking. We decided to go with faith, instead of prognosis. We did everything we could in the way of treatment, and left it in God's hands to say when this fight was over."

Eighteen months after Michael's initial diagnosis, it

became clear that the treatments were not working and his cancer would take his life soon. Michael decided that he wanted to have one last trip with his family, so he and Erin took the children to Walt Disney World. "He wanted them to have one more really great trip to remember," she says. Three months after they returned, Michael Stennis lost his fight with colon cancer and died.

But Erin says the work has not. "The response has been tremendous. You know there is a ripple effect. And by what we've gone through, we have been able to effect change for other black men and women. People who didn't know about this disease before know about it now and are getting tested—earlier." Erin says that many men in their church family have gone in for screenings and found precancerous polyps. "One of our deacons says that Michael's example saved his own life. Without colon cancer hitting so close to home, he would have never gone on his own steam," she says. Because of their experience, many of her friends have insisted that their husbands and fathers get screened, as well. "Something powerful has come out of our sadness," she says.

"The last few words Michael said to me were, 'Slow down.' And right along with that he said, 'Keep fighting,'" she says. And she is.

As you can see from Erin's struggles with Michael, getting black men to go to the doctor to get screened for colorectal cancer is an extremely difficult task. Yolandra Johnson, MD, is a nationally known gastroenterologist. "Many of the black men I see come in because someone else—usually his wife or significant other—has been in and urged him to go," she says.

Colorectal cancer, which is cancer that affects both

the colon and rectum, if left undiagnosed is one of the top cancer killers in the United States. Nearly 8,000 black men get a new colorectal cancer diagnosis each year. And approximately 3,400 black men die annually from the disease, mostly because they don't get screened or treated until the cancer is in its advanced stages. We don't do a lot of talk about colorectal cancer in our community, but Erin will tell you that it is one of the most important conversations you can have with someone you love. It's the third leading cancer death among both black men and black women. It is alarming and particularly unfortunate because Dr. Yolandra Johnson says that colorectal cancer is one of the truly preventable cancers.

While the numbers of deaths from colorectal cancers is dropping on a national level, the number of diagnoses and deaths in our black communities has not dropped to the same extent that it has among whites.

Black men and black women are equally as likely to develop colorectal cancer. And because this cancer is often found in its later stages in people of color, both have poorer survival rates. But that could be changed dramatically if we got over our fears and got screened and treated.

Pat Smith can also give testimony as to the importance of early detection and screening. Her husband, Julius, lost his long battle with advanced colorectal cancer in 2006. "I could have gotten diagnosed sooner, but I didn't pay attention to the things my body was saying to me," Julius said. It was a difficult road for Julius, but Pat was at his side supporting him in his journey all the way. "I'd tell anybody who will listen to go get screened—the earlier, the better," Julius said before he died.

What Are the Warning Signs?

- A change in bowel habits
- Diarrhea, constipation, or feeling that the bowel cannot empty completely
- Blood (either bright red or very dark) in the stool
- Stools that are narrower than usual
- General abdominal discomfort (frequent gas pains, bloating, fullness, and/or cramps)
- Weight loss with no known reason
- Constant tiredness
- Nausea and vomiting

Note: *Remember, early colorectal cancers do not usually cause pain. So don't wait until he experiences pain to get help.*

How Does His Heath History Affect His Risks?

Having a personal history of colorectal polyps, which are extra tissue that grows in the intestine, can put him at an increased risk for colorectal cancer. Most polyps are not cancerous, but over time they can become malignant if they are not removed. Also having a history of chronic irritable bowel syndrome can raise his risk, along with ulcerative colitis, which is a disease that causes ulcers and sores in the lining of the rectum and colon.

What Role Does Family History Play?

The American Cancer Society says that somewhere between 5 and 10 percent of colorectal cancer is caused by an inherited gene. Another 20 percent of all people who have colorectal cancer have two other family members who have had the disease. So we know that some families are at higher risk.

The problem in black families is that this is not the kind of information usually shared. So many of us don't really know what cancers run in our families, because the "C" word has always been taboo. That's one of the reasons why collecting family health history information now and talking openly and honestly about what is going on with our health can be a gift today and to future generations.

Screening and Diagnosis

The American Cancer Society recommends that men and women begin getting annual screenings for colorectal cancer starting at age fifty if there are no other symptoms, warning signs, or a family health history of the disease. But the American College of Gastroenterology suggests that black men and black women may develop colon polyps at a younger age than white persons, and now recommends that they begin getting screened at age forty-five.

While Dr. Johnson and other experts in the field are not sure what causes colon cancer among blacks, she does suggest that perhaps black men and black women die from the disease more often because of the lateness in which they get screened and diagnosed, like Michael.

Experts used to say that screening should start with a fecal occult test that looks for blood in the stool. You can get this test from your doctor, or you can buy one at the drug store and either mail it in or take it back to your doctor. But Dr. Johnson suggests that a colonoscopy be the first line of screening for black men and black women starting at age forty-five. She suggests that black men (and black women) have a colonoscopy every ten years if their previous colonoscopies were negative and they have no other major risk factors.

What Is a Colonoscopy?

If you ever watch the *Today* show, you've seen colonoscopy become famous when then anchor Katie Couric had one on national television. It is the gold standard at this point for diagnosing colorectal cancer. Colonoscopy enables your doctor to thoroughly examine the lining of your colon (large intestine) for abnormalities and polyps. He or she will insert a flexible tube as thick as your finger into your anus and slowly advance it into the rectum and colon. The beauty of a colonoscopy over the other options is the tube not only has a camera that allows the doctor to see your colon, it also has a pair of nippers at its end that allows him or her to snip off any polyps to have them biopsied.

Polyps are abnormal growths in the colon lining that are usually not cancerous. They can be anywhere from the size of a tiny dot to several inches. Because your doctor can't always tell a benign polyp from a cancerous one, he or she might send removed polyps for analysis. Because cancer begins in polyps, removing them is an important means of preventing colorectal cancer.

Colonoscopy is well tolerated and rarely causes much pain. Your man might feel pressure, bloating, or cramping during the procedure. His doctor might give him a sedative to help him relax and better tolerate any discomfort.

The colonoscopy is a fairly quick procedure. It usually takes fifteen to sixty minutes. After the colonoscopy, the doctor will explain the results of the procedure and what he or she saw. It will usually take a few days to get back the results of the biopsies. Your man will need to have someone with him to drive him home from the procedure.

His doctor will give him instructions and dietary restrictions to follow and what cleansing routine to use for the day and night before the procedure. Usually this involves drinking a special colon cleansing solution or clear liquids and special oral laxatives. The colon must be completely clean for the procedure to be accurate and complete. So you will need to make sure to help him follow his doctor's instructions carefully.

Does Insurance Cover Screening?

Although specialists are recommending that black men be screened at earlier ages, the current recommended age accepted by most insurance companies is age fifty unless the person is considered to be at high risk or has had some of the warning signs, such as blood in the stool. Although specialists are recommending that black men be screened at earlier ages . . .

- Most private insurance and Medicare will cover the cost of a fecal occult blood test, which is about $10 to $15, for a person over fifty every year.
- Most private insurance will cover the cost of a flexible sigmoidoscopy screening for men over age fifty every four or five years. Medicare will pay 80 percent of the fee, which averages $150 to 300, for a person over fifty, every four years.
- The coverage of the cost of a colonoscopy, which is the most specific of the three screening tests, varies from insurance carrier to carrier. Check with your provider in advance of a test. Medicare will cover 80 percent of the cost of a colonoscopy, which is about $800 to $1,600, for a person over fifty every ten years.

What He Should Do If He Gets a Colon Cancer Diagnosis . . .

If his polyps or tumors are found to be cancerous, Dr. Johnson says his medical team will "stage" his disease, which means that they will tell him how advanced his disease is and what kinds of treatment will be used.

At Stage 0, the colon cancer is at its most treatable stage. The cancer has not grown beyond the intestinal lining or the rectum. Most often, the removal of the polyps is all the treatment that is needed.

If the cancer is Stage I, the tumor has grown into the layers of the lining of the rectum, but has not spread beyond the rectal lining. The cancer is usually surgically removed and many patients need no further treatment.

If the cancer is Stage II, the tumor has grown through the wall of the rectum into nearby tissue. It has not yet spread to the lymph nodes. Stage II rectal cancers are usually treated by surgery along with both chemotherapy and radiation therapy.

If the cancer is Stage III, it has spread to nearby lymph nodes but not to other parts of your body. The doctors will usually perform surgery and radiation therapy will be given before or after surgery.

The best approach to colorectal cancer is to stop it in its tracks through screening and through paying attention to the warning signs.

GERD Can Lead to Cancer

Gastroesophageal reflux disease (GERD) causes food or liquid in the stomach to back up into the esophagus. The food is acidic because it is partially digested, and therefore irritates the esophagus. It causes acid indigestion and heartburn. Black men have a high rate of GERD and are at risk for Barrett's esophagus, a precancerous condition that damages the lining of the esophagus and can lead to esophageal or throat cancer.

If a man is experiencing regular bouts of heartburn and acid reflux, or using over-the-counter antacids for an extended period of time, he should talk to his physician. A doctor can work with him on diet and lifestyle changes, as well as prescribe medications that can quiet heartburn and heal his throat and reduce his risk of esophageal cancer. If he has been experiencing untreated acid reflux or GERD for a long time, his doctor may refer him to a gastroen-terologist for an endoscopy or a biopsy to make sure that no precancerous or cancerous conditions exist.

BREAST CANCER

Elmer Edwards and his wife, Imogene, have always been healthy and active. He keeps a healthy weight and, pays attention to warning signs that may mean that he needs to get some things in check. So imagine his surprise when he got hit with the one-two punch of cancer. He was diagnosed with breast cancer and then prostate cancer. Fortunately, with Imogene's help and support, Elmer made a full recovery.

Breast cancer in men is rare, but it does happen. Out of the new breast cancer diagnoses in 2005, only 1,700 of those were men. Many people do not realize that men have breast tissue and that they can develop breast cancer.

Like all cells of the body, a man's breast duct cells can undergo cancerous changes. Because women have many more breast cells than men do and perhaps because their breast cells are constantly exposed to the growth-promoting effects of female hormones, breast cancer is much more common in women.

Early detection improves the chances that male breast cancer can be treated successfully. Many men's breast cancers could have been found earlier by their health care professional if they had regular checkups. Although there are many similarities between breast cancer in men and women, several important differences affect early detection. The most obvious difference between the male and female breast is size. Because men have very little breast tissue, it is easier for men and their health care professionals to feel small masses.

On the other hand, because men have so little breast tissue, cancers do not need to grow very far to reach the skin covering the breast or the muscles underneath the breast. Therefore, although male breast cancers tend to be slightly smaller than female breast cancers when they are first found, they have more often spread beyond the breast. The extent of spread beyond the breast is the most important factor in the prognosis (outlook for chances of survival) of a breast cancer.

Some men ignore breast lumps or attribute them to an infection or some other cause, and they do not get medical treatment until the mass has grown significantly. Also, some men who think breast lumps occur only in women are embarrassed about finding one and worry that someone might question their masculinity. This attitude may also delay diagnosis and reduce a man's odds for successful treatment.

Because the male breast is much smaller than the female breast, all male breast cancers start relatively close to the nipple, so spreading to the nipple is more likely.

Treatment is often the same as it is for women. The options are surgery, then radiation, chemotherapy, or a combination of the two. Like breast cancer in women, the earlier a man is diagnosed, the better his prognosis.

SKIN CANCER

Although it is one of the few cancers that is much rarer in black men than it is in white men, it is important to be aware that black men do get skin cancer. And like many cancers, because of lack of prevention, screening, and early detection and treatment, skin cancers in black men and black women can be deadly. But they don't have to be. Skin cancers are absolutely preventable if you are armed with good information and put that knowledge to use.

According to Marcy Street, MD, a dermatologist who specializes in skin cancer surgery, the most common form of skin cancer among blacks is melanoma, a cancerous growth that begins in the skin cells that produce skin coloring. She says that black skin is loaded with a large amount of melanin—the pigment-producing substance that gives us color and helps to provide some protection from the sun's damaging effects. But it doesn't provide complete protection. Dr. Street urges all her patients no matter what their ethnicity to wear protective sunscreens to give extra protection against skin cancer. A study from the American Academy of Dermatology reports that once the disease has been diagnosed, African Americans have higher death rates from melanoma than other racial groups, including fair-skinned whites, mostly because of later detection and treatment.

It's important to note that skin cancer in blacks may not appear on the areas of the skin that are exposed to the sun. Unlike whites whose cancers typically show up on the face, chest, and back, melanomas in blacks most often are found in mucous membranes of the mouth, genitals, or nasal passages and between toes and fingers. Black men and women don't normally associate the appearance of unusual growths with skin cancer. Instead, we ignore them—a deadly mistake.

Screening

With a 96 percent successful cure rate, skin cancer is one of the easiest cancers to treat when detected before it spreads to the lymph nodes and to other parts of the body. Undetected, only about half of African Americans diagnosed with skin cancer survive the disease. Dr. Street suggests setting up an appointment for the men in your life at least once a year with your family practice physician or with a dermatologist for a screening for suspicious moles or lesions on the body and extremities. "Women also need to be helping the men in their lives pay attention to moles and sores that don't heal, change shape or color or size, which may be a warning sign of a precancerous growth."

Even after his screening visit in the doctor's office, at least once a month make sure to have him look on the palms of his hands, between his fingers and toes, in his genital area, and on the soles of his feet for suspicious growths. "These are some of the primary areas that men of color are developing precancerous lesions and moles," Dr. Street says. By going in to see a medical professional early, he can have any precancerous moles and lesions that look like sores that do not heal treated, before a cancer that is more difficult to treat, or requires surgery, can occur. When looking at the skin for possible skin cancers think about the ABCDs. "The A is for asymmetry, the B is for the irregular border around the suspicious area, the C is for the color of the area, which is often dark or black, and D is for diameter and change in the size of the diameter in the area," Dr. Street says.

Prevention

Dr. Street says the best way for people of color to protect themselves is to develop the habit of wearing sunscreen with an SPF rating of 15 or more. You can find the SPF on the packaging of any tanning product. The sunscreen helps to protect the skin from harmful ultraviolet rays of the sun, causing burning and other damage. She suggests that families apply sunscreen every day, and reapply every couple of hours, if you are going to be outside in the sun, in the park, or on the beach. "Pick up some extra to put in his gym bag or golf bag, too," she adds.

CLINICAL TRIALS

Throughout this book, there is a lot of information on the numbers of black men who are affected by all the major diseases including cancer. But there is a gap of knowledge in knowing why they are so adversely affected and in the development of effective treatments for men of color.

A medical research team in Detroit at Wayne State did a review of the medical records of 175 black and 252 non-black lung cancer patients. They looked at a number of indicators, such as sex, age, socioeconomic status, insurance type, and disease stage. They found that the black patients were significantly less likely to participate in the studies.

Black men and black women are still extremely skeptical about being involved in these studies for many reasons, including concerns about the quality of care. But experts say that the quality of care is actually higher. "When you go into a clinical trial, you have twenty experts in your particular cancer, and the doctor who's involved in clinical studies will likely be the better doctor," says Dr. Otis Brawley, a cancer expert at the Winship Cancer Institute at Emory University School of Medicine. Dr. Brawley conducts clinical studies and examines why some patients enroll and others do not.

Myths and mistrust are sometimes associated with clinical trials, particularly for many black men. The unethical treatment of blacks enrolled in the Tuskegee Syphilis Study where penicillin treatment was withheld resulted in years of mistrust toward doctors, health care, and anything that has "study" attached to it. In order to understand why, you have to go back and understand the horror of Tuskegee. In that 1932 study, about 400 poor black men with syphilis in Macon County, Alabama, were allowed to die so researchers could study the effects of the disease. The story is recounted in the HBO movie *Miss Evers' Boys*, starring Alfre Woodard. This could never happen today, thanks to laws and restrictions that prohibit unethical practices in clinical trials.

Why Should He Participate?

New medicines and cures are being developed based on clinical trials. Medicines work differently in different groups. In general, new medicines are not being developed with black men in mind. The medicines that black men take for prostate cancer or lung cancer have not been as well tested for those men, because they don't generally participate in clinical trials.

What Does He Need to Do to Enroll in a Clinical Trial?

The first step to getting into a clinical trial is talking with the doctor about trials that are currently open for new patients. Also take the time to investigate some of the Web sites that we list in the resources section. Work with your medical team to find out the best way to further pursue a study.

But understand that just because he is willing to participate doesn't mean that the man in your life will be accepted. Before joining a clinical trial, a man must qualify for the study. Some research studies seek participants with illnesses or conditions to be studied in the clinical trial, while others need healthy participants. If he's not accepted, he shouldn't take it personally. All clinical trials have guidelines about who can participate. The factors that allow someone to participate in a clinical trial are called "inclusion criteria" and those that disallow someone from participating are called "exclusion criteria." These criteria are used to identify appropriate participants and keep them safe, and to help ensure that researchers will be able to answer the questions they plan to study.

The criteria are based on such factors as age, gender, the type and stage of a disease, previous treatment history, and other medical conditions.

There is a lot of information on current clinical trials on the Internet. Check out www.clinicaltrials.gov. Each study has its own benefits, including, in some cases, free health care while in the study. Make sure he understands all the terms and benefits of the study before signing on.

What Happens During a Clinical Trial?

The clinical trial process depends on the kind of trial being conducted. The clinical trial team includes doctors and nurses as well as social workers and other health care professionals. They check the health of the participant at the beginning of the trial, give specific instructions for participating in the trial, monitor the participant carefully during the trial, and stay in touch after the trial is completed.

Some clinical trials involve more tests and doctor visits than the participant would normally have for an illness or a condition. For all types of trials, the participant works with a research team. Clinical trial participation is most successful when the protocol is carefully followed and there is frequent contact with the research staff.

What Is Informed Consent?

Informed consent is what helps protect the man in your life in a way that Tuskegee did not protect those 400 black men. During informed consent, a man is informed of all the key facts about the particular clinical trial before he decides whether or not to participate.

Informed consent is not a one-shot deal. It is also a continuing process throughout the study to provide information for participants. To help someone decide whether or not to participate, the doctors and nurses involved in the trial explain the details of the study. Then the research team provides a document that includes details about the study, such as its purpose, duration, required procedures, and key contacts. Risks and potential benefits are explained in the informed consent document. The participant then decides whether or not to sign the document. Informed consent is not a contract, and the participant may withdraw from the trial at any time.

Thinking About a Clinical Trial?

Suggest that he consider the following questions and discuss the answers with his doctor as he make his decision on participation:

- What is the purpose of the study?
- Who is going to be in the study?
- Why do researchers believe the experimental treatment being tested may be effective? Has it been tested before?
- What kinds of tests and experimental treatments are involved?
- How do the possible risks, side effects, and benefits in the study compare with his current treatment?
- How might this trial affect his daily life?
- How long will the trial last?
- Will hospitalization be required?
- Who will pay for the experimental treatment?
- Will he be reimbursed for other expenses such as travel or meals?
- What type of long-term follow-up care is part of this study?
- How will he know that the experimental treatment is working? Will results of the trials be provided to him?
- Who will be in charge of his care?
- Is he risking his life by forgoing traditional treatment to go with the experimental trial?

Clinical trials may not be for everyone, but they do offer many terrific opportunities for many men.

CHAPTER 10

Mental Health

If there is a true silent killer among men of color, it is probably undiagnosed and untreated mental health issues. Black men simply don't talk about their mental health and wellness. If you start talking about the subjects that we address in this chapter, like depression, bipolar disorder, anxiety, and anger issues, then you start to step all over their culture, religion, and their masculinity.

Black men who live with mental health issues are often a part of a very secret society. According to the Black Mental Health Alliance, 7 percent of all black men will develop some form of short- or long-term depression during their lifetime. The number is probably larger because so many black men do not have access to screening and treatment and go unreported as a result. The Alliance also suggests that only a small percentage of blacks who were depressed said they had ever gone to a mental health specialist.

Statistics show that black men are less likely to be treated with medications for their depression and other mental illnesses such as bipolar disease, than white men. There are many reasons for this. One is the unwillingness to seek out help, another is the community stigma that still exists around mental health.

The medical profession is now understanding and embracing the role that mental health, or lack of it, plays in the overall health and well-being of black men, and is starting to make some inroads into identifying problems that patients might be having. When black men experience depression, they may present symptoms differently—with anger and irritability instead of the sadness that is normally associated with it. That anger or irritability could be misinterpreted as the stereotypical "angry black male."

The medical community acknowledges that there is often a link between the physical and mental well-being of a man. Laura Mathew-Thompson is the chair of the Family Medicine Committee of the National Medical Association, and a black family practice physician in North Carolina. She says that many times she can pick up on the first signs of depression in the men in her office. If a male patient of hers comes in because of lack of appetite, inability to sleep, or sleeping too much, it signals to her to look deeper than these symptoms, to the common underlying causes of mental health issues.

In this chapter, we will talk about mental health, specifically depression, anxiety, and bipolar disease, and ways that black women can begin to look at mental health as a part of the overall health of the men they love.

Mary Hall-Thiam had only been married a year when depression became a real part of her life and her marriage. "My husband was teaching school in Detroit, but the pressures of the issues that the children come to school with and the lack of support from the school system seemed to push him over the edge," Mary says.

She says they spent a lot of time talking about what was going on at school, but she had no idea that it was affecting him in such a deep and profound way. "He was having trouble sleeping, at first. Then he started crying out in the middle of the night."

She says that his sadness and anger got so bad that she was afraid to leave him alone. "I took time off work, because I was really afraid that he would do something to himself." It was a very stressful time for both of them.

"That's when I knew that we were in trouble and we needed to seek out some help." But like most black men, going anywhere for "help" was not on his radar. She really had to do some work to convince him to go. Getting him into care was even more difficult, because he is from Nigeria, and in his culture, you just don't go outside for help.

Mary helped her husband find a therapist that he trusted. And their work together uncovered something surprising. His depression and anxiety were triggered by working in what was a "war zone" atmosphere. Mary says that his symptoms were that of someone who had post-traumatic stress disorder (PTSD), not unlike the kind experienced by veterans of war. Often, people with

PTSD have persistent frightening thoughts and memories of their ordeal and feel emotionally numb. PTSD was first brought to public attention by war veterans, but it can result from any number of traumatic incidents, including difficult work environments.

One of the solutions Mary's husband came up with was to remove himself from that stress, for his own health and well-being. He is now in a new education environment and doing well. But Mary attributes the fact that together they went for help as the main reason for the positive outcome.

The Black Mental Health Alliance for Education and Consultation and Community Voices released a report on black men and mental health called *The Souls of Black Men* in 2003, based on the discussions among a group of black men they called upon to talk openly about their thoughts on and experiences with mental health. Their candid responses were heartbreaking and frightening. One man that they interviewed said, "No black man in America is ever mentally healthy." Another said, "Who really gives a damn about the black man in America."

That man is right to a certain extent, because there is so little talk within our community about the things that plague our men. Sadly, it was a tragic headline that recently put the national spotlight on depression in black men. In 2005, James Dungy, eighteen-year-old son of NFL coach Tony Dungy, committed suicide. After overdosing on prescription pills a few months before his death, he told police he was depressed. It was almost unfathomable that a young black man with a future so bright would take his own life. Yet it is on the rise. The rate of suicides among young black men, between the ages of fifteen and nineteen, from 1980 to 1995 rose 146 percent. How could this happen? Where was the help?

When we look away in silence we are dooming our black men in ways that we can't imagine. Studies show that black men who are not treated for their mental illnesses are more likely to become incarcerated, homeless, substance abusers, and victims of homicide and suicide.

WHEN THE STIGMA OUTWEIGHS THE PROBLEM

Annelle Primm, MD, is the director of minority and national affairs for the American Psychiatric Association and an associate professor of psychiatry at Johns Hopkins University. Dr. Primm says that the role of our values is just one piece of the puzzle. She and many others say black men don't face up to depression due to the stigma of being mentally ill or emotionally not well.

Alvin Poussaint, MD and professor of psychiatry at Harvard Medical School, is the co-author with Amy Alexander of *Lay My Burden Down,* a book that traces the issue of black men and depression and suicide. In his book, Dr. Poussaint says that psychologists and psychiatrists have to pay attention to those types of behaviors and look at them in a context in the same way they would look at someone who, in fact, was depressed or maybe suicidal.

Another issue is the lack of black psychiatrists and psychologists in this country. "We know that people of color are vastly under-represented among all healing professions, and blacks make up only 2 percent of psychologists and psychiatrists and 4 percent of social workers," Dr. Primm says. "Black men are reluctant to seek out help anyway, but they are often uncomfortable talking to non-black professionals about mental health issues.

"Being a black man in America has a major impact on people's psyche. There are micro-insults and then there are macro-insults: not being able to get a cab, not being able to get decent employment or education," Dr Primm says of the things that contribute to mental illness in our communities. "People of color, and African Americans in particular, are exposed to racism. There is a direct impact on mental health and physical health, like with high blood pressure," Dr. Primm says.

John Head is the author of *Standing in the Shadows: Black Men and Depression*, an honest and unflinching look at black men and depression from the inside out. John is an award-winning journalist, but he also is a black man who has struggled in silence for years with his own demons of depression. "From my own experience with depression," John says, "early intervention would have been any intervention at all."

"For more than 20 years, I didn't understand what I was going through. So I did nothing about it," John says. Over the years John says he had episodes of going down emotionally and coming back up and then going down again. As time went by, the down periods got deeper and longer, the up periods got shorter. "If you think you can just let it go on and you'll snap out of it eventually, that's not the way it works," he says.

Major depression accounts for up to 35 percent of

suicides. "The link between depression and suicide is so strong because depression robs you of hope. You reach a point where you believe life is not worth living, and you believe suicide is the only way out. Imagine what it's like if this is the way you feel all the time," John says.

Unfortunately, that's what it's like for many young black males. They don't see a future for themselves. They can't see the value of their own lives. That puts them at greater risk of suicide, according to John.

He says that the real numbers of suicide in our communities may be even larger than we suspect. "There is a general reluctance to admit that a death is the result of suicide. This attitude is even stronger among African Americans. Also, some kinds of self-killing—such as 'suicide by cop' or slow suicide through drug abuse—are not counted as suicides," he says.

The weight of depression can be so real, especially if it has no name, and a man thinks there is no hope or cure for what's going on. John says that he has done his own dance with the ultimate complication of depression—suicide. "I stepped back from the brink of suicide because I realized I had reasons to live. The primary reasons were my sons. I grew up without a father in the home. When I thought about how much worse it would be for my sons if they not only had to live without me, but also had to deal with the fact that I took my own life, I knew I couldn't do that to them," John says.

As black women and as members of communities, we have a strong responsibility to change the lens by which people view depression and other mental illnesses.

Black people are finally learning to stop stigmatizing their grandmother's diabetes or their father's high blood pressure. We know that these are "real illnesses." Mental illnesses among our black men must be looked upon the same way.

Some warning signs of depression and mental illness are:

- Inability to carry on basic tasks
- Staying in bed all the time
- Can't concentrate or remember things
- Loss of appetite
- No interest in activities that used to bring him pleasure, such as sports, going out with friends
- Loss of sexual desire
- Trouble falling asleep or staying asleep
- Weight loss or gain
- Unexplained anger
- More drinking and drug use

Dr. Mathew-Thompson says that "as women, we really need to look at the underlying anger that our men seem to experience and act out on."

She urges women to support the men in their lives in getting a diagnosis and treatment. Like Mary and her husband, we have to be willing to trust in help. What often happens is that once a person enters into treatment, the family will say, "Oh, there's nothing wrong with you, just get yourself together." That can sometimes discourage a man from continuing treatment. Black women must be more vigilant in creating a safe space for the men in their lives to be open about their feelings, and in encouraging their quest for needed sustained support.

Dr. Primm suggests that communities include in their health fairs mental health screenings by trained professionals. Then once a man has been diagnosed, we need to make sure that he has access to mental health support from a clinical social worker who has trained in depression, a psychologist, psychiatrist, or psychotherapist. "We also need to make sure that men are given resources on where to get help whether they have insurance or not," Dr. Primm says.

The best way to begin seeking out a mental health resource is probably through the family practice doctor. That doctor can refer you to a mental health provider that he or she knows and trusts.

Of course, one of the obstacles to care for many black men is lack of health coverage for mental health services. Many private practice psychiatrists and psychologists will only see private pay or insured patients. One way to find out about free resources is to call your local health department. Although they may have large waiting lists, many health departments do offer mental health services. They can also connect you to hospital-based support groups and other community services. There are free hotlines and sometimes mental health resources available in community centers and churches. There are also free support groups, where people who have gone through the same sort of situation can come together. Be persistent both in finding help and persuading the man in your life to go for help.

John cautions black women not to look for a quick fix. Coming out of depression and other mental illness can be a lifelong struggle for some black men. But experts agree that getting into some form of treatment is key. The treatment may consist of regular visits with a mental health professional as well as some form of prescription medication designed to address a man's particular mental health issue.

Mothers, daughters, sisters, and lovers all need to be prepared to help with follow-through. It is not uncommon for a man to receive a mental illness diagnosis and never seek treatment, or begin treatment for a while then stop. Another problem is getting a man to stay on prescribed medications that can help him control his mental illness. Compliance with taking the medications is a huge issue. The man is probably resistant to taking medications anyway, and there may be real or perceived side effects, such as feeling drowsy, foggy, or even more unbalanced initially. And many men, as soon as they start to feel the slightest bit better, stop. When they stop, their depression or anxiety may return, putting them back in the same spot they started.

They commonly self-medicate with alcohol and street drugs rather than to take the prescriptions on a long-term basis. Some men who suffer from bipolar disease say that the medications take away the highs and just leave them with the lows.

Many people go through short-term bouts of depression that may be related to a situation, such as a divorce, grief, or job loss. But mental health issues don't always go away quickly. Some, such as clinical depression, bipolar disorder, and post-traumatic stress, can require lifelong awareness and commitment on the part of the man and the people who love and support him in his struggles. As one man told us, "Being mentally well is an everyday decision, and an everyday struggle. I will have to work to be healthy every day of my life."

But it doesn't have to be that way. The first step is to acknowledge mental health issues as illnesses that require medical treatment, in the same way that other chronic conditions, such as diabetes, do. The next step is to seek out help through mental health practitioners, including psychiatrists, psychologists, and community mental health programs. Practitioners can do an assessment to determine just what mental illness the person is suffering from and create a treatment plan combination for each individual's needs. Some men are able to control their condition through prescription medications, and others are able to do so through a combination of therapy and medication.

Depression is often treated with medications such as Paxil, Prozac, Wellbutrin, and Zoloft, to name a few. In addition, a man may attend therapy sessions with a mental health provider. There are also some lifestyle changes that can make a big difference for a man suffering from depression. Exercise, eating a healthy balanced diet, developing hobbies and interests are all important tools in a man managing his depression. Women can be of tremendous support to a man who is suffering with depression by encouraging him to seek out help and follow his treatment plan.

THE SPIRAL INTO OTHER RISKY BEHAVIORS

Black men with mental illnesses are at high risk of developing substance-abuse problems. John says that our communities are a breeding ground for the cycle of substance abuse and other risky behaviors that continue to feed depression. "Unfortunately, in African American communities in poverty, there is a proliferation of liquor stores and a very high availability of illegal drugs," John says.

"When people are intoxicated from alcohol and other substances, they do things that they normally wouldn't do. And that brings on additional untoward consequences, like violence, incarceration, further health problems. Maybe they have unprotected sex or share needles, which increases their risk for diseases like HIV/AIDS and hepatitis," John says.

He and Dr. Primm agree that all of these activities combine to increase risk for unemployment, for homelessness, and those situations, in turn, just reinforce the mental health problems. "If we could identify early and treat psychological distress, perhaps we could prevent a lot of deaths due to substance use, a lot of lives wasted in prisons, and optimize the health and well-being and quality of life in our communities."

BIPOLAR DISORDER OR MANIC-DEPRESSIVE ILLNESS

Bipolar disorder, also known as manic-depressive illness, is a serious medical illness that affects many black men. The illness can cause shifts in a person's mood, energy, and ability to function. A person who has bipolar disorder suffers through dramatic mood swings from overly "high" (manic) to sad and hopeless (depressive), and then back again, often with periods of normal mood in between. The periods of highs and lows are called episodes of mania and depression. The swing can result in damaged relationships, poor job or school performance, and even suicide.

Bipolar disorder typically develops in late adolescence or early adulthood. It is often not recognized as an illness, and a man can suffer for years before it is properly diagnosed and treated. Like diabetes or heart disease, bipolar disorder is a long-term illness that must be carefully managed throughout a person's life.

What Are the Symptoms of Bipolar Disorder?

Signs and symptoms of *mania* (or a *manic episode*) include:

- Increased energy, activity, and restlessness
- Excessively "high," overly good, euphoric mood
- Extreme irritability

- Racing thoughts and talking very fast, jumping from one idea to another
- Poor concentration
- Little sleep needed
- Unrealistic, exaggerated beliefs in one's abilities and powers
- Poor judgment
- Spending sprees
- A lasting period of unusual behavior
- Increased sexual drive
- Abuse of drugs, particularly cocaine, alcohol, and sleeping medications

Signs and symptoms of *depression* (or a *depressive episode*) include:

- Lasting sad, anxious, or empty moods
- Feelings of hopelessness or pessimism
- Feelings of guilt, worthlessness, or helplessness
- Loss of interest or pleasure in activities that were once enjoyed, including sex
- Decreased energy, an overall feeling of fatigue or of being "slowed down"
- Difficulty concentrating, remembering, having a hard time making decisions
- Restlessness or irritability
- Sleeping too much, or inability to sleep
- Change in appetite and/or unintended weight loss or gain
- Thoughts of death or suicide, or even suicide attempts

Diagnosis of Bipolar Disorder

Like other mental illnesses, there is no blood test or brain scan that can tell if a man is suffering from bipolar disorder. Mental health experts make their diagnosis of bipolar disorder through talking to the person, reviewing symptoms and the cycle of symptoms, and reviewing the family history.

Treatment

People tend to struggle with bipolar disease throughout their lives. Because bipolar disorder is an ongoing illness, a man has to make a commitment to long-term treatment, which can include medication and psychosocial treatment, if he is going to be successful in managing his symptoms over time.

In most cases, bipolar disorder is much better controlled if treatment is continuous than if it is on and off. But even when a man is taking his meds continuously, he can still have setbacks in mood changes and behavior. The key is to be aware of those changes and check in with his doctor or therapist right away. By reporting changes early, he may be able to work with his doctor to prevent a major episode. Managing bipolar disorder, just like other mental illnesses, is a partnership.

Medications

Medications for bipolar disorder are prescribed by psychiatrists with expertise in the diagnosis and treatment of mental disorders. While primary care physicians who do not specialize in psychiatry may also prescribe these medications, it is recommended that people with bipolar disorder see a psychiatrist or go to a mental health center for treatment.

Lithium is often very effective in controlling mania and preventing the recurrence of both manic and depressive episodes. Anticonvulsant medications, such as Depakote or Tegretol, can have mood-stabilizing effects and may be especially useful for difficult-to-treat bipolar episodes. Newer medications, including Lamictal, Neurontin, and Topamax, are being studied to determine how well they work in stabilizing mood cycles. A man should talk to his health care provider about which medications will work for him.

CHAPTER 11

Oral Health

We spend so much time worrying about the health care "biggies," but pay little attention to our oral health. It is important to address because poor oral health can lead to infections of the gums that can spread through the whole body, as well as other illnesses. This chapter takes a look at the importance of oral health in our black men, and how they can prevent tooth loss, gum disease, and other health ailments that come from poor oral health.

A painful tooth or gum abscess, for example, can lead to missed days at work. But the links between poor oral health and heart disease are strong, too. Since we've already talked about how good our men can be at ignoring the signals that their bodies give them, it's no surprise that they aren't paying proper attention to their teeth and gums either. Pain that they can no longer bear is the main reason that men report going to a dentist. Prevention is not high on the list.

The biggest reason that black men don't seek out a dentist is the lack of dental coverage and/or the lack of money to pay for services. Dental care often places low on the priority list. If money is tight because your man is trying to keep food on the table, and the lights and heat on, a dental visit is one of the first things to get scratched off the health care to-do list.

Finding a dentist is not always easy, either, and getting scheduled in a timely manner can be hard because of the shortage of dentists in some areas.

IT STARTS WHEN THEY ARE YOUNG . . .

In 2000, while he was United States surgeon general, Dr. David Satcher released a report on oral health in America. The report points out that people of color including black men have poorer oral health than other groups, and that tone for dental health is set when they are children. Our black preschoolers have one and a half times more tooth decay than white children, according to the CDC. As mothers, we need to start teaching our sons and our daughters the importance of dental health in our overall health. We need to make a commitment to getting our children to the dentist early to start laying the groundwork for a lifetime of great oral health.

Over a third of our young black children get insufficient care for their oral health problems including tooth decay. Many black children have not been trained in the basics of oral health such as brushing and flossing. But we have the opportunity today to make sure that our little boys and our little girls understand the importance of a healthy mouth and strong teeth.

AND IT GETS WORSE . . .

Gum disease develops when plaque builds up around the teeth and gums. Plaque contains bacteria and toxins that can irritate and inflame the gums. In its early stages, gum disease is called gingivitis, which is signaled by gums that bleed after brushing and flossing. If left untreated, it becomes the more serious periodontitis. Although gum disease is mostly linked to poor oral hygiene, some people have a genetic predisposition to this condition. Black adults have 30 percent more gum disease than white adults. The National Cancer Institute statistics say that black men have the highest rates of all oral and pharyngeal cancers of any group. Did you know that 34 percent of black seniors have lost some or all of their teeth to gum disease?

This is troubling by itself, but it is also a concern because poor oral health is linked to other health conditions such as heart attack and stroke. The American Heart Association says that people with gum disease that comes from plaque are more likely to also have plaque buildup in their arteries (artherosclerosis). This condition causes narrowing of the blood vessels, which can lead to heart attack or stroke. Michael Roizen, MD, the author of the book *Real Age*, says that improved oral health including flossing can reduce a man's risks for heart disease and add years to his life.

Most black Americans don't go to the dentist with the regularity that they should. Nearly half of all white Americans have gone to the dentist for either prevention or treatment of some aspect of their dental health in the past year. According to the CDC, only 27 percent of blacks have been to visit the dentist in the last year.

Each year black men make the decision to ignore a toothache unless it is causing them such pain that it affects their ability to carry on their duties and responsibilities. If we can get them to act on tooth and gum pain sooner, they could protect themselves from losing teeth and gum tissue. If we could persuade them to see a dentist, they could also be screened earlier for oral cancers.

Ruthie Jimerson, DDS, is a dentist who does nothing but extractions and providing dentures. Her busy practice is full of patients who come in to have their teeth pulled because they are damaged beyond anything a regular dentist can do for them. Dr. Jimerson says that black women need to start scheduling regular dental checkups for our young boys and men and continue to impress upon them the importance of their oral health.

She recommends finding a dentist who is good with children, and understands their fears, which will result in not being afraid of going to the dentist the rest of their life. Some men are truly traumatized by the idea of their regular cleanings and avoid them like the plague.

Many black men are taking their teeth for granted. They think they will always be there, no matter how much they neglect brushing, flossing, regular cleanings and exams, and treatment, Dr. Jimerson says.

"When they neglect their mouths and their teeth fall out or have to be taken out, they are surprised," she says. It's sad because like many of the health issues that black men face, tooth loss and gum disease are preventable.

Not only is neglecting their oral health a surefire ticket to cavities and gum disease, but it is also thought to contribute to heart disease and stroke. Also, dentists see a link between gum disease and lack of control of insulin levels in diabetic patients.

TIPS FOR GREAT ORAL HEALTH

- Encourage him to brush his teeth at least twice a day and to floss regularly. The most common cause for bad breath, in addition to tooth loss, is poor dental hygiene.
- Discourage his intake of surgary drinks and foods, or at least have him brush immediately after drinking or eating them.
- For boys and young men who are playing sports, make sure they have and wear a mouthguard that fits. Having a mouthguard not only helps to protect against knocked out teeth during a game, but it also helps to prevent injuries such as broken jaws, concussions, and neck injuries.
- Continue to encourage him to stop smoking or using other tobacco products that can affect the appearance of his teeth.

WHEN SHOULD HE SEE THE DENTIST?

You may need to help the men in your life find a dentist and schedule regular visits for exams and cleanings. To keep cavities and gum disease at bay, a man should see a dentist at least twice a year. If he already has gum disease, his dentist may want him to come in for cleanings once every three or four months, to keep plaque and tartar down.

And beyond the routine cleanings and checkups, remind him when he needs to see his dentist right away. The following symptoms call for immediate attention:

- Gums that bleed when he brushes or flosses
- Swollen, puffy, red, or tender gums
- Constant bad breath—a sign of tooth decay or gum infection, too
- Teeth that are loose or are falling out
- Changes in the bite or the way his teeth fit together when he bites
- Signs of a toothache
- Tooth or gum sensitivity to hot and/or cold foods and drinks
- Any unexplained jaw pain

WHAT HE SHOULD BE DOING AT HOME . . .

Here are some key things that every man who is taking his oral health seriously should be doing:

- Brushing after every meal or at least twice a day
- Flossing at least once a day using a dental floss that does not shed or shred
- Using a toothpaste that has fluoride included to help to protect the teeth
- Replacing his toothbrush once every three or four months because they wear out
- Replacing his toothbrush after a cold or the flu
- Eating apples, carrots, and high-fiber greens. They are good for the teeth. Cranberries are thought to help prevent gum disease and plaque, too.

CHAPTER 12

Let's Talk About Sex

Sex and sexuality are a normal and healthy part of a man's life. His sexual health and well-being are probably very important to him. We can't really talk about him being the most healthy person that he can be without talking about issues around his sex life. There are many things that affect a man's sexual well-being, including his overall health.

When a man goes into a doctor's office to discuss problems in the bedroom, lack of desire, or other issues, most physicians will look at his overall health. They will perhaps do a complete physical on him, run some blood work, and talk to him about stresses in his life. The elements are interconnected.

This chapter deals with two important issues in the sexual health of black men: erectile dysfunction and sexually transmitted diseases (STDs), including

HIV/AIDS, which is now an epidemic in communities of color. Use it as an opportunity to open the lines of communication with your husband, lover, father, son, or friend. Some of the information in this chapter can be a lifesaver for him and even for you.

ERECTILE DYSFUNCTION

Impotence or erectile dysfunction (ED) is bound to happen to a man at some stage in his life. In this section, we will talk about what we all know can be a very sensitive subject. The causes, and the possible solutions, include prescription medications. Many men (and their partners) suffer unnecessarily for years because they won't seek out the help that is available.

The older a man gets, the more likely he is to have a bout of ED. By the time they hit their forties, about 5 percent of all men experience it. Twenty-five percent of men age sixty-five will have experienced some form of ED. It is an interesting note that we could talk to men about every health issue except this one when we researched this book. No man seems to want to admit on the record that he has or has ever had any kind of performance issues.

What Is It?

In order to explain erectile dysfunction, let's explain how a man's plumbing really works. When a man becomes sexually aroused, the brain sends a message that causes blood to rush to his penis. If for some reason, say circulation problems or an enlarged prostate, blood flow is restricted to the penis, the man cannot get an erection. Although he might act like it is the worst thing that has ever happened in his life, or that he is the only man this has happened to, it is very common.

Dr. Terry Mason, a urologist who is also the author of *Making Love Again: Renewing Intimacy and Helping Your Man Overcome Impotence,* says that 30 million American men experience ED at one time or another, according to the National Institutes of Health. There are a lot of reasons for ED; some of them are physical and some of them are what's going on in his head at the time, or a combination of the two, Dr. Mason says.

The occasional problem is not really what frustrates men or causes problems. It is the chronic complete impotence, partial or brief erections that cause a man to seek out help from a medical professional. The chronic ED can be very frustrating for any man. It causes problems with self-esteem and can put a strain on relationships.

What Causes ED?

Over half of the cases of ED are side effects of diseases such as diabetes, atherosclerosis (hardening of the arteries), and kidney disease. It is estimated that up to half of all men with diabetes have ED at one time or another.

We know that black men suffer disproportionately with diabetes, so we know that this is a potential problem for our black men. High blood pressure and high cholesterol can also affect sexual function in men. Unfortunately, ED is one of the reasons that many black men suddenly stop taking their blood pressure medicine. Instead of deciding to stop taking the medication cold-turkey, which is common, Dr. Mason suggests that men come back in to make modifications in their prescriptions. Oftentimes adjustments to his prescriptions will prevent ED.

In addition to medicines designed to lower blood pressure, there are over 200 other medications that can affect a man's sexual function. For example, heart medications, tranquilizers, sedatives, and anti-depressant medications can also cause ED.

Figuring It Out . . .

If he is having a problem that won't seem to go away, encourage him to make an appointment with his doctor. Dr. Mason suggests this should be sooner rather than later. There is a lot of anxiety that goes with ED. If an office visit can get to the root of the problem, he will be a lot happier.

At his appointment, his doctor will probably run some blood tests, including checking his hormone levels, blood sugar, liver and kidney function, cholesterol levels, and thyroid function. A complete blood count (CBC) will eliminate the possibility that anemia is causing the problem. The doctor will also probably run a urinalysis looking for unusual levels of protein, sugar, and testosterone that could point to diabetes, kidney problems, or a testosterone deficiency.

To narrow down the problem even further, the doctors may order an ultrasound to make sure there is no scarring or blocking of blood flow. A digital rectal examination will determine if he has an enlarged prostate gland that is blocking blood flow and nerve impulses to the penis.

It doesn't sound very romantic, does it? But these are some of the ways that medical experts can get answers to what's going on. Once they have a diagnosis, then they can figure out a course of treatment. One of those options is oral medications, called enzyme inhibitors, like Viagra, Levitra, or Cialis. If the doctor prescribes these medicines to him, he will need to take them once a day. If your man has had a heart attack or stroke in the last six months, or if he is taking heart medications to treat chest pain or a class of drugs called alpha-blockers used to treat high blood pressure and some non-cancerous prostate problems, then he should not be taking enzyme inhibitors. And he should never use any of these medicines without being under a doctor's supervision, which means he should also never use someone else's meds for ED.

Some men, who wished not to go on the record with suffering from ED, did tell us that these drugs can be miracle workers. But one added, "Not all the problems are physical, and a medicine like this helps with the physical. Sometimes you gotta get into your heart and your head if you want to solve some of those problems."

How Much Is Too Much?

Whatever the course of treatment that he and his doctor settle upon, you need to help him make sure that he takes exactly what is prescribed. Sometimes men get the idea that if one pill will work, two will work *really* well. That is not a good plan. These are strong medicines and taken in the wrong dosages, or with other medicines, they can be dangerous.

Prevention

There are many reasons why a man will experience temporary erectile dysfunction. Some are preventable. He can decrease the likelihood if he:

• limits or avoids alcohol or drug use.
• stops smoking (there it is again).
• exercises routinely.
• reduces the amount of stress in his life.
• gets plenty of rest.
• deals with any issues around depression.

What Else Can You Do?

Probably the best thing you can do is discuss it with him, but don't make a big deal of it. He will probably be doing enough worrying about it for the both of you. Don't personalize it. ED is not a sign of diminished sexual desire for you. ED is not your fault. It does not mean that you are not attractive to him.

He really shouldn't have to deal with the stresses of ED and the stresses of reassuring you, too. Keep the lines of communication open so that he feels comfortable talking to you about what he's thinking and going through. In many cases, ED is situational or temporary, but in other cases, depending on the causes (other medications, cancer, etc.), a couple may need to keep the lines of communication open with their health care provider. With a little patience, a lot of understanding, and a good doctor's help, this too shall pass.

ED

Some medical conditions such as diabetes and hypertension are known to cause erectile dysfunction. But there are other causes that may be as close as your medicine cabinet. Not all of these medications cause ED in every single patient, but there are over 200 prescription medications and other over-the-counter meds known to cause ED in some men. If the man in your life is experiencing symptoms of ED, one of the first places that doctors look for clues is the medications he is taking. If it is being caused by his medications, both prescription and over-the-counter, he should work with his doctor on substituting other medications with fewer side effects.

Here are a few common culprits:

- Tranquilizers
- Some medications, including some of the diuretics, used to manage high blood pressure (Maxzide, Lasix, Lopressor)
- Anti-depression medications (Prozac, Zoloft, Elavil)
- Amphetamines
- Cancer medication (Eulexin, Lupron, Myerlan, Cytoxan)
- Antihistamines used to treat stuffy noses and congested chests with a cold or flu (Dramamine, Benadryl)
- Heartburn and acid reflux medications (Tagamet)
- Sleep medications (Sonata, Ambien)

Remember also, tobacco use, excessive alcohol use, marijuana, cocaine, and other substances have been known to negatively affect sexual performance, especially if used over time.

HIV AND AIDS

HIV/AIDS is taking a major toll in our black communities. Black people make up approximately 13 percent of the U.S. population, but they make up over half of the numbers of Americans living with HIV/AIDS. Statistics reveal that 40 percent to 50 percent of all men living with HIV/AIDS are black. Even though the media does not report on HIV/AIDS in this country the way it did in the late 1980s and early '90s, this monster still kills. It is the leading cause of death for blacks who are between ages twenty-five and forty-four.

"Young, handsome, talented, and with all the potential in the world." That's how Frankie Travis describes her son, Arthur, who lost his battle with AIDS in 2000. Unlike many mothers who struggle with their son's sexuality, Frankie says she never missed a beat. "He was my baby and I loved and still love him."

She says that when he contracted the virus, he was determined to do what he had to in order to fight the disease, and she was determined to do whatever she had to do to give him love and support and make him healthy again. Arthur's sister Debbie Cuzean says that is exactly what her mother did. "She was his caregiver until the end."

Frankie says that women who have sons who are gay or are dealing with their sexuality need to offer their love and support, no matter what. "Arthur knew he could come to me with anything," Frankie says. The virus brought that message home to her, and many other mothers who have lost their sons to this disease.

There are thousands of mothers and fathers, sisters and brothers who have a story like Frankie's. HIV/AIDS touches every aspect of our community, not just our men. Among new diagnoses, 71 percent are women. And sadly 70 percent of all new diagnoses of children with HIV/AIDS are our black babies who are getting it at birth through infected pregnant mothers.

What Is HIV/AIDS?

HIV is human immunodeficiency virus. AIDS is the acquired immunodeficiency virus. HIV is not an easy disease to get. You can't get it from being in the same room with someone who has the HIV/AIDS virus. You won't get it by touching someone with the virus. The virus is transmitted through blood, semen, vaginal fluids, and breast milk.

Amadou Diagne, MD, an AIDS researcher, says, "A man can have the HIV virus, or be HIV-positive without having AIDS, but if a man has AIDS, he definitely has HIV. There is a six-week marker after a person has been exposed to accurately tell if he is positive for HIV or AIDS. Even then, the virus can lay dormant for years or decades before becoming AIDS." Dr. Diagne says that thanks to the variety of medications now available, many men and women are living with HIV, and it is not turning into AIDS.

Some people who are HIV-positive have symptoms that look and feel like a flu or a cold. Sometimes a person will have fever, headache, swollen lymph nodes, and a sore throat. Sometimes a person who has contracted the virus has no initial symptoms, but is still diagnosed through an HIV/AIDS test.

HIV is contracted most commonly through unprotected sex, if one of the two has the HIV/AIDS virus. But the virus can also be passed through IV drug users sharing needles. And although it is rarer now, you may remember that tennis great Arthur Ashe died of AIDS, after contracting the virus through a blood transfusion from blood infected with the virus.

Still, it needs to be said again and again, that the most common means of spreading the disease in our black community is through unprotected vaginal, anal, and oral sexual contact. Dr. Diagne says that latex condoms have helped reduce the numbers of infections through sexual contact, but they do not provide 100 percent protection. Half of all male infections came from men having sex with other men. But 80 percent of black women get the virus through sex with a male.

Diagnosis

Dr. Diagne says that it is important for a black man to know his HIV status, especially if he has had multiple partners. "He should get tested. It is a simple blood test, and it is strictly confidential." A person can also buy an oral test, where you can swab the lining of the mouth, wait thirty minutes, and get the test results. The oral tests, which are 99 percent accurate for detecting the HIV antibody but not the HIV virus, and which can be purchased online or in pharmacies, should still be confirmed by a blood test.

Even though the HIV virus becomes active in the body within days or weeks, the current tests detect HIV antibodies in the blood, which can often take months to build up. So oftentimes having an HIV test right after exposure will give a negative test result for the HIV antibodies simply because the antibodies have not had enough time to build up yet. The test should be repeated again six months later.

There are free HIV/AIDS testing and counseling centers in many cities and on college campuses. By law the results are kept confidential. Most clinics require that a person come back to get his or her results. If he or she is found to be HIV-positive, he or she is given information on and links to treatment options.

Prevention

The best prevention is abstinence. If there is no sexual contact (oral, anal, or vaginal), there is no risk of contracting the virus sexually. Another method of prevention is both partners getting tested before having sex and remaining monogamous. The best protection for sexually active individuals is the use of a latex condom each and every time a person has a sexual encounter, whether it is homosexual or heterosexual activity. Although no means of protection is 100 percent short of abstinence, condom use offers some protection even if one partner is infected.

Greg Millett, an epidemiologist in HIV/AIDS at the Centers for Disease Control, says there is a lot of education being done in terms of prevention, but we still have much to do. There is evidence that there is low condom use among black couples, which is thought to be lower than white couples.

Prison and HIV/AIDS

We haven't even begun to address the role of prisons and incarceration in the epidemic among people of color. HIV/AIDS is alive and well in prisons all around the country, through men having sex with men and through IV drug use. These are men who are not given condoms in prison and they are also men who are being released out in the community with no means for consistent treatment. They come back to their neighborhoods, homes, families, and women and have unprotected sex. Some do not know their HIV status; others choose not to disclose it to their sexual partners.

Can HIV/AIDS Be Treated?

Let us say right up front that there is no cure for HIV/AIDS. Up until 1987, when AZT, the first drug that showed hope, was introduced, there were no really effective treatments that kept the disease at bay. It was the age of the death sentence. If you got HIV, you were going to get AIDS and you were going to die. Ask any gay man who lived through the first wave of the epidemic.

Dr. Robert Washington is one of those men. "I suspected I had the disease for a while, but it wasn't confirmed until I was tested in the late '80s." Dr. Washington says that he luckily lived with the virus for over thirteen years before getting on any kind of treatment program. "The main reason, at first, was because there was no treatment at the time I was diagnosed." Robert says that the fact that he wasn't fully out of the closet was also a barrier to seeking medical attention. "But I also have to say that I was lucky. Many people during that time period died. I think that it helped that after I was diagnosed, I never had unprotected sex, which probably kept me from re-infecting myself with a more virulent strain of the disease," he says.

AZT, an anti-HIV medication that works to reduce the amount of the virus in the body, changed everything for a large number of people living with the disease. It kept people healthier longer, but it had high side effects for many men who took the medication. Sometimes the side effects were worse than the virus.

The world of treatment for a person living with HIV/AIDS keeps evolving. The drugs that have had the most success are called antiretroviral therapy or cocktails, which are very potent combinations of other drugs, and help a person living with HIV stay healthy. But the medicines are often expensive, often with side effects that make living with the disease sometimes unbearable. Some medications, such as protease inhibitors, and neucleoside/neucleotide reverse transcriptase inhibitors, can cause a host of side effects including diarrhea, kidney and liver failure, heart attack and stroke, and pancreatitis.

One of the problems with the medications has been getting people of color to comply 100 percent, even if they are fortunate enough to be able to afford or access them. Having had to switch treatments several times because of side effects and bad reactions, Dr. Washington says that we need to be careful in placing blame when it comes to compliance. "There are many reasons why a person might not comply. Many of the side effects can make a person under treatment sicker than the disease itself," he says.

Many people stop taking the meds because of these side effects. They do so without consulting a physician or having the doctor replace current medications with another drug with fewer side effects or adding other medications that can diminish side effects. Dr. Diagne urges against this. He says, "Taking the drugs erratically is almost as bad as never taking the drugs at all."

When we talk about compliance with a doctor's recommendation we must also look at the fact that only 14 percent of black people who need these medications have any kind of health insurance. The medications are very expensive, sometimes amounting to several hundred to thousands of dollars a month in prescription bills. Fortunately many state public health programs are working with local AIDS action groups and clinics to make medications and treatment available to those who need them.

There is no cure for HIV or AIDS, but it doesn't have to be a death sentence. The medical community is racing toward finding a vaccine or a cure for the virus, but at this point, there is no magic bullet. However there has been progress in keeping people healthier and living longer. Many people living with the virus have been doing so for decades. They take their meds and are monitored by doctors, but they have also found ways to not let the disease define them. In fact, Dr. Washington says that it was his work with a young man who had found out that he had been infected, and struggled with being forsaken by his black church, that led him to become a minister himself.

Pernessa Seale runs the New York–based HIV/AIDS service organization the Balm in Gilead, which partners with black churches to provide HIV/AIDS services. Pernessa has been a trailblazer in the fight against HIV/AIDS—a black woman who saw what was happening in her community and went into action mode. "We saw how, in the early days churches were closing their doors, not wanting to deal with people with HIV/AIDS," says Pernessa. Today, Seale says, "We work with about 10,000 churches around the country." Faith communities of color have different levels of commitment, Seale notes, but they're finally asking, "What can we do for people with disease?"

That's what we black women have to do. We have to fight this disease on all fronts. We have to fight it in our bedrooms, at our dinner tables, in our churches, on our streets. It means forgetting about the how, if the how makes you uncomfortable, and get down to the who. The who is all of us.

The best protection from HIV and other STDs is abstinence. If you are not having sex, you are not at risk for contracting the disease from sexual contact. But we all know that this may not be realistic. What is realistic and has been shown to be the best ammunition in the fight against HIV is latex condom use and HIV testing. Never have unprotected sex with a man until both of you have had an HIV/AIDS test.

One of the hardest conversations that a black woman may ever have with the man in her life, whether it is her boyfriend, husband, or longtime companion, is the condom talk. Black women are often reluctant to push the issue, but Gary Bell, the executive director of Philadelphia-based Blacks Educating Blacks on Sexual Health Issues (BEBASHI), says that it is up to us to protect ourselves. "Men have a lot of reasons why they don't want to use a condom," Bell says. He also says that none of them are valid. Experts say that women must be prepared to walk away. Or as they say, "No glove, no love."

Bell regularly conducts workshops with black women that include developing and practicing the skills to insist upon condom use. He says that although it sounds easy, it is hard to get women to take a stand on self-protection. Data from the CDC's sex survey supports Bell's observation: Only 32 percent of black women ages fifteen to forty-five reported using condoms the last time they had sex.

"Getting a woman to assume responsibility for protecting herself starts with valuing herself," Bell says. "A woman should be able to stand up for that value and say, 'I'm not going to let anybody poison it.'"

What About the Down Low?

Thanks to J. L. King, every black woman between eight and eighty knows what the "down low" is, or so they think they do. His book *On the Down Low* addressed something that has always existed in our community, and in everybody else's, too—men who secretly have sex with men, and hide it from the women they are also having sex with. It is, as King describes it, a secret society, and his book was a deadly blow to already fragile relationships between black men and black women.

Keith Boykin is an openly gay man who has challenged King's theories about black men on the down low and its impact on the numbers of black women who are infected with HIV or are living with AIDS. Boykin says that as he tours speaking about his book, *The Myth of the Down Low,* black women aren't asking how to protect themselves against HIV. Instead, he says, "They are telling me that they now assume that every man they meet is on the down low. They even have down low detective Web sites out there." Rather than looking for someone to blame, we all need to put the focus back on personal responsibility to protect ourselves.

Maisha Drayton, an HIV/AIDS outreach worker in Buffalo, New York, says, "We all have to do everything we can to protect ourselves from the risks of HIV infection, no matter where the risk comes from."

We also need the skills to respond to the gameplaying and half-truths many brothers dish out. Bell says that when asked to wear a condom many men will respond, "I'm not gay" or "I had a HIV test six months ago."

When it comes to sex, there are risks we know and risks we can never be certain of. Remember that we carry a sexual history that is not just ours but that of every person we've been with and every person they've been with. So the first line of defense against HIV infection for black women is not interrogating a man about the down low but insisting on condom use and testing, no matter what.

Tips for Women in the Fight Against HIV/AIDS

- Start talking about condom use early in the relationship, that is, if you are planning on taking the relationship to the next level. The best time to start having the conversation about using a condom is when you first see the relationship going in the direction of sexual intimacy.
- Test together. Testing and knowing your HIV status is one important tool in further preventing the spread of the disease.
- Stick to your guns. Say, "No love without the glove," and mean it.
- Keep some condoms ready to go, in case he says, "I would but I don't have any on me."
- Be clear that asking your partner to use a condom is not questioning his sexuality. It's about protecting both of you.
- Consider getting and using the female condom, which is a sheath that fits inside the vagina to prevent pregnancy and STDs. You can excuse yourself and slip it in. It has been proven to be very effective if used correctly and consistently. You don't need his consent, and in most cases, your partner won't even know you are using it. You can pick up a package of female condoms in most places that sell male latex condoms.

- Know the facts. No, the condom is not too small (as many men will say). Gary Bell says that he has put condoms over his elbow to demonstrate to women that the average condom does fit most men. And they do come in different sizes.
- Be clear about your own self-worth and what you are willing to do to protect it.
- Know the importance of HIV/AIDS testing. Never have unprotected sex without testing.
- Above all, be prepared to walk away. If he isn't prepared to protect your life and his, he probably isn't someone who has your back in other situations.

The Realities for Black Women

Yes, ladies, romance, intimacy, and commitment are important to us in our relationships with our men. We want to be talked to and understood, and be shown some genuine affection. Studies show that the "warm-up" is just as important to us as the act itself is to our men. But things have changed a lot over the past twenty years.

We now worry not only about making him talk to us and treat us special, but in the era of HIV/AIDS and other STDs, we also worry about protecting ourselves and them. Many of you who are reading this are thinking that we just have to be talking to someone else. And maybe we are, but in a book about men's health and the health of our communities we felt that it was important to give you some food for thought:

- More than 40 percent of men who are sexually active with three or more partners still never use condoms, even with all the information out there about the spread of HIV/AIDS.
- Surveys say that 40 percent of men who have a primary sexual relationship (wife, girlfriend) *and* a secondary partner will wear a condom with the secondary partner. Ladies, this means that 60 percent are not using a condom.
- We talk a lot about HIV/AIDS, but other sexually transmitted diseases are equally as real. They may not be as life threatening as HIV/AIDS but they have their own dangers.
- We have the highest rate of STDs (outside of HIV/AIDS) in the free world.
- The statistics are staggering. There are approximately 100,000 new diagnoses of HIV/AIDS in this country each year (men having sex with men, men and women of all ethnicities).
- HIV among older Americans is on the rise. At least 30,000 men and women who are forty-five and older are HIV-positive or living with AIDS. Not all of the men were categorized as MSM (men having sex with men) or IV drug users. Some 30 percent of the Americans who have been diagnosed with HIV/AIDS considered themselves to be heterosexual.

Having a talk with a partner or potential partner about using a condom may feel like throwing a bucket of cold water on intimacy. But it is that fear and reluctance that is spreading HIV/AIDS like wildfire in our communities.

OTHER SEXUALLY TRANSMITTED DISEASES

The United States has the highest rates of STDs of any country in the industrialized world. Some men are aware that they have or have had a sexually transmitted disease, but many have no idea that they are a victim. As with HIV, the best protection against other STDs is abstinence. The next best thing is latex condom use, each and every time a man has sex.

The number of men and women infected with HIV each year is staggering, especially in the black community, but the number of people who will be diagnosed with an STD also deserves our attention. This year:

- There will be approximately 34,000 new syphilis infections.
- At least 877,000 people will contract chlamydia.
- There will be over 300,000 new cases of gonorrhea.
- And surprisingly, there are 45 million men and women living with herpes from sexual contact.

Do we have your attention yet?

Types of STDs

There are many types of sexually transmitted diseases. The best way to prevent them is through regularly using condoms and limiting the number of sexual partners. Sexual contact should be avoided any time there is a questionable symptom or genital sore present to keep from spreading the disease to other partners. Usually if an STD is present, both partners will need to be treated to prevent re-infection.

Chlamydia

The incidence of chlamydial infections is three times that of gonorrhea and thirty times that of syphilis. This bacteria can cause symptoms of burning during urination, pelvic inflammatory disease (PID), vaginal or penile discharge, or no symptoms at all. Many men will have no noticeable symptoms, or symptoms so mild they go unnoticed. Infertility can result from chlamydia if it is not diagnosed and treated.

If either partner is diagnosed with chlamydia, he or she must receive antibiotic treatment even if there are no symptoms present. They must avoid intercourse until treatment is completed. If left untreated, chlamydia can cause permanent damage to reproductive organs and potentially render a person sterile. Complications in pregnancy can occur and newborns (infected by the mother's birth canal) can have severe enough infections to cause death.

Gonorrhea

Often referred to as the "clap," gonorrhea has symptoms that include penile discharge, painful urination, and testicular or abdominal pain (and some who have gonorrhea have no symptoms). The infection may also enter the bloodstream, becoming widespread, resulting in infection of joints, skin, heart, liver, and central nervous system. Those symptoms usually begin two to six days after exposure to the bacteria. Infection of the anal canal and throat are common as a result of oral and anal sex when one of the partners is infected. Symptoms of anal infection include anal burning, itching, pain, and discharge. Infection of the throat may result in soreness with puss-like material visible on the tonsils, or back of the throat, but occurs very often without symptoms or lesions.

Gonorrhea cannot be diagnosed by a urinalysis. Special tests must be done in order to detect the bacterial organism responsible for the disease. Antibiotic treatment varies depending upon where the infection is located. Treatment requires antibiotics for both partners as well as a follow-up test to be sure the organism is no longer present.

Herpes

Herpes is transmitted to a partner during oral or genital sexual contact. It can also be transmitted through skin-to-skin contact, such as kissing when one of the parties has a herpes lesion. Once the virus enters your body, an active infection may develop. If it does, you may be capable of passing the virus to another person. This virus causes blister-like sores on or near the genitals, mouth, or other parts of the body. The sores are usually painful or itch, but sometimes symptoms are so mild that the virus is transmitted unknowingly.

Following an initial outbreak, some people have recurrent outbreaks of herpes sores, usually during times of stress. A herpes simplex infection appears two to twenty days after exposure. It takes the form of sores on or around the lips, mouth, or face; or sores in or around sex organs in the case of genital herpes. These sores may itch, burn, or be quite painful. They may be accompanied by swollen glands, general muscle aches, and fever. In genital herpes, a burning on urination in both men and women or mild vaginal discharge for women may be experienced. Initially the sores may last for a few weeks and then heal completely.

The virus, however, remains in your body, but enters a dormant phase. Some new herpes patients never experience a second episode following the initial infection. Among those who do, some experience recurrences only infrequently, others quite regularly. Recurrences tend to be less severe than the initial infection. General health and resistance, physical trauma, and emotional stress may be factors involved in a recurrent outbreak of sores.

Genital herpes is contagious just before and throughout the entire time any sign of an active outbreak persists. When any sign of a recurrence is noticed (itching, burning, tingling, or sores), you should prevent the affected area from coming in contact with another person. It also means not engaging in oral to oral contact or oral to genital contact.

Herpes symptoms can often be confused with other diseases. See a doctor right away for an accurate diagnosis and early treatment. There is no cure. Treatment includes prescription antiviral medications, such as Zovirax, Famvir, and Valtrex, which can help decrease symptoms and shorten the duration of the herpes outbreak. But the herpes virus will always remain dormant in the body. Personal hygiene is very important if you are diagnosed with herpes. Touching a sore and then touching some other part of your body can move the virus to a new location. This is especially true during the early stages of the disease.

Genital Warts

Genital warts are caused by the human papilloma virus or HPV. The virus can cause bumpy growths around the vulva and anus or on the penis and scrotum. They often appear clustered, like cauliflower, or are sometimes too small to see. Without the appearance of warts, there may not be any other symptoms. Some types of wart virus are associated with the development of abnormal cell growth, which may progress to the growth of cancerous cells. Men and women with genital warts or exposure to a partner with warts should be tested by a doctor.

Genital warts can be transmitted via skin-to-skin contact. Warts can occur on the penis, scrotum, vulva, vagina, cervix, anus or, rarely, on the mouth or throat. Studies indicate HPV may affect up to 70 percent of sexually active people, most of whom will never develop warts or any other changes caused by this virus.

However, concern arises because HPV is linked to increased risk of cervical cancer in women.

Condoms, while essential in preventing most sexually transmitted infections, have limited value in preventing HPV. This is because the virus involves the entire genital area and can be spread by skin-to-skin contact.

Treatment of genital warts is similar in both sexes, with local applications of podophyllin or trichloroacetic acid, or by freezing the warts with liquid nitrogen weekly until warts disappear. Severe or very persistent cases may require longer therapy or surgical removal. As with all treatments, the exact mode is determined by each person's needs.

Syphilis

Syphilis is a disease that is usually sexually transmitted. It most commonly occurs in men and women between twenty and twenty-four years old. Symptoms of syphilis vary according to the stage of development of the illness. Initially, a painless sore, called a canker, can develop. Cankers are usually located on the external genitalia, anal canal, or mouth, but may occur on any area of the body. Several weeks or months later flulike symptoms and rash may occur, and then disappear. If undetected and untreated, syphilis can cause damage to the infected person's nervous and cardiovascular systems. There are four stages of syphilis: primary, secondary, latent, and late stage.

Primary syphilis is characterized by a canker that occurs approximately twenty-one days after contact and usually heals within six weeks, even without medication. Enlargement of lymph nodes located in the groin, armpits, and neck usually occurs within one week of appearance of the canker.

Signs of secondary syphilis begin to appear six weeks to six months after contact. This stage is characterized by lesions of the skin. The skin rash that occurs ranges from flat to raised to blisterlike lesions. These lesions occur on the palms of the hands, soles of the feet, face, and scalp. The raised lesions may break down in moist areas of skin folds to form broad gray-white or pink lesions. With secondary syphilis you may also have fever, weight loss, and loss of appetite. The symptoms of this stage of syphilis go away without treatment, but it does not mean the disease is gone. In fact, without treatment, the disease will progress to more serious stages.

Latent syphilis is the next stage of infection. Lab tests can confirm whether a person is positive for syphilis, but there are no outward signs of infection at this stage. Latent syphilis can last for many years and is followed by late syphilis or a slow destruction or breakdown of functioning in the central nervous system and blood vessels, particularly the aorta, in 30 percent to 50 percent of untreated patients.

Blood tests are more commonly used to diagnose the disease, but syphilis cannot be detected this way until four to six weeks after the appearance of a canker. The best treatment for syphilis is injection of penicillin. If left untreated it can eventually result in permanent organ damage and even death.

Hepatitis B

Hepatitis B is a virus that can be passed through body fluids during sex and is extremely contagious. Each year 40,000 new infections are diagnosed, and 75 percent of all cases occur among fifteen- to thirty-nine-year-olds. It is thought to be 100 times more infectious than HIV (the virus that causes AIDS). This virus causes inflammation of the liver, which can become chronic (lifelong), and it has also been associated with cancer of the liver.

Hepatitis B is found in all types of body fluids including semen, blood, and saliva. It can stay alive on contaminated surfaces for as long as a month. This means that you can contract this viral infection through an open wound, even a small cut, just by touching a contaminated surface in a restroom, locker room, or kitchen.

You can also contract the virus directly from an infected person through obtaining cuts and scrapes during sports, kissing, having unprotected sex, and sharing personal items like tweezers, razors, toothbrushes, or earrings. Contaminated instruments for body piercing or tattooing can also harbor the virus.

Of the people who contract hepatitis B, 50 percent demonstrate no symptoms. The others may have flulike symptoms, such as fever, fatigue, muscle or joint pain, and loss of appetite and/or vomiting. Jaundice, yellow discoloration of the skin and eyes, is a key sign of hepatitis.

Prevention rests on immunization. Get him to ask his doctor about making sure that he has had a hepatitis B vaccination, which offers immunity to 90 percent of healthy adults, or the necessary booster shots, during his next physical or routine office visit.

WHAT DO WE TELL OUR TEENS?

We know beyond a shadow of a doubt that teens are having sex. Not all teens. Not necessarily your teens. But the data is clear. Our jobs, as parents of young black males, is tough anyway, but is even tougher when you talk about sex. It used to be that we worried about unplanned pregnancies. Now we worry about that plus AIDS, which could end their lives, or other STDs that could leave them sterile in the future.

We can tell you that parents who have specific religious and moral values regarding sex face a real dilemma in discussions with our teens. Your religion and your values may say that you firmly teach your children abstinence until marriage. Of course, as a parent, it is important to give your children consistent messages that will help to shape their moral fiber.

But one of the problems that researchers are seeing is that the abstinence-only message may prolong the period before a teen has sex for the first time (by months or up to a year), but it makes them more vulnerable when they do make the decision to have sex (without your permission, we are sure). One recent teen sex study shows that once teens who are abstinent for some time begin having sex, they are more at risk for unplanned pregnancy and/or STDs because they did not have correct information on prevention.

So here is the cold hard decision you have to make as a parent. How do you temper your values with the information that will protect your sons (and daughters) from all the dangers that are out there? It can feel like you are damned if you do, and damned if you don't.

The good news is that almost all the literature shows that giving teens information about sex and how to protect themselves is not going to make them go out immediately and do it. And you can also arm them with information on how to avoid peer pressure, how to get out of tricky situations, and how to keep his values front and center. It's all part of the package.

Let's look at it another way. As a parent I have a choice of providing my son with accurate, well-researched information about sex—including protecting himself and the responsibilities that go with having sex. I get to tell him about the benefits of waiting. I get to tell him about the threat of HIV/AIDS. I get to tell him that he does not have to prove his manhood by putting himself at risk.

Or I can choose to not tell him anything. I can give him one option (an option that in reality is not ours to give unless we put them under house arrest). When we know better, we do better—and we know that "Just Say No" never worked in communities of color (or anywhere else). If I take that option, here is the other scary thing I can count on. He is going to get the information somewhere. Others who do not necessarily have my values and my belief systems are going to give him their take on it, and he may make a different, uninformed decision as a result.

CHAPTER 13

Aging

There are some natural progressions that can come with getting older, such as thinning hair, eyesight that isn't what it used to be, and perhaps some diminished hearing. Many of the illnesses and conditions that settle in as we age have already been discussed. But there are a few that bear your attention in helping to manage a black man's health. This chapter addresses two of the most difficult parts of the aging process: arthritis and Alzheimer's disease.

WHAT IS ARTHRITIS?

Arthritis is one of the most common chronic conditions among Americans today, especially among those over fifty. Nearly 66 million people live with some form of arthritis and the pain that can go with it. Arthritis is having a major impact on our men. It is one of the leading causes of work-related disability, second only to heart disease. While black men have nearly the same incidence of arthritis as white men, they are more likely to have physical limitations and severe joint pain. Black men may be disabled by the disease due to lack of access to the health care system, or a reluctance to seek out care and medication that can help them manage this very painful group of diseases. A black man living with arthritis may have a hard time walking, dressing, or even bathing as the disease progresses.

The word "arthritis" literally means joint inflammation. Arthritis is a general name, but there are nearly 100 different forms of the disease. Different forms of arthritis can affect different age groups and can affect men and women differently. These different forms can cause symptoms such as moderate to severe joint pain, stiffness, and swelling in joints and other supporting structures of the body such as muscles, tendons, ligaments, and bones. Some forms can also affect other parts of the body, including various internal organs. Men should make sure they talk about their symptoms with their primary care physician to help get diagnosed and treated. More advanced arthritis sufferers may seek out help from a rheumatologist, an internal medicine physician who specifically treats arthritis.

Some more common types of arthritis are:

- *Osteoarthritis.* A degenerative joint disease in which the cartilage that covers the ends of bones in the joint literally deteriorates, causing pain and loss of movement as bone begins to rub against bone. It is the most common form of arthritis, and tends to become worse with age. It can be controlled with over-the-counter medications such as acetaminophen or other pain relievers such as Celebrex, Aleve, and ibuprofen that can help to temporarily reduce the swelling in the joints.

- *Rheumatoid arthritis.* An autoimmune disease in which the joint lining becomes inflamed as part of the body's immune system activity. It affects women two to three times more frequently than it does men.

- *Gout.* Affecting mostly men, this is another extremely painful condition that most often attacks the small joints of the body, especially the big toe. Fortunately, gout almost always can be completely controlled with medications such as nonsteroidal anti-inflammatory (NSAIDS) drugs and changes in diet. Persons taking medications for gout should be monitored regularly by their health care provider.

There is no cure for arthritis, but much is being done to manage its progression and the pain that can go with it over time. Many black men live in constant pain due to their arthritis because they refuse to seek medical attention or follow the tips doctors offer to help manage the disease.

But there are things that can be done to successfully manage arthritis and its pain. Tell him to check with his health care provider before using any of these methods.

Short-term solutions include:

- *Moist heat.* Supply this with warm towels, hot packs, warm paraffin wax dips, a bath, or a shower. Used at home for fifteen to twenty minutes three times a day this can help relieve symptoms. Ask your health professional about treatments that use short waves, microwaves, and ultrasound to deliver deep heat to non-inflamed joint areas to increase circulation. Deep heat is often used around the shoulder to relax tight tendons prior to stretching exercises, and can provide temporary relief.

- *Cold.* Supply with a bag of ice or frozen vegetables wrapped in a towel. This helps to stop pain and reduce swelling when used for ten to fifteen minutes at a time. It is often used for extremely inflamed and tender joints and can be more effective and appropriate in this situation than deep heat.

- *Hydrotherapy.* Water therapy can decrease pain and stiffness. Exercising in a large pool may be easier because water takes some weight off painful joints. Community centers, YMCAs, and YWCAs have water exercise classes developed for people with arthritis. Some patients also find relief from the heat and movement provided by a whirlpool.

- *Mobilization therapies.* Include traction (gentle, steady pulling), massage, and manipulation (using the hands to restore normal movement to stiff joints). When done by a trained professional, such as a certified massage or physical therapist, these methods can help control pain and increase joint motion and muscle and tendon flexibility.

- *TENS and biofeedback.* Transcutaneous electrical nerve stimulation and biofeedback are two additional methods that may provide some pain relief, but many patients find that they cost too much money and take too much time. In TENS, a mild electrical shock is transmitted through electrodes placed on the skin's surface.

• *Relaxation therapy.* This type of therapy also helps reduce pain. A physical therapist or massage therapist can teach a man how to release the tension in his muscles to relieve pain in the painful area, at home. The Arthritis Foundation has a self-help course that includes relaxation therapy.

Medications

In addition to these methods, the physician can work with the man in your life to decide on medications that may help him manage his arthritis pain and symptoms.

The physician's decision on which medications should be used depends on many things, including desired health outcome. If a man is simply trying to reduce the amount of pain, his physician may suggest that he use one type of drug. But if he is trying to reduce the amount of inflammation in the joints, he may be given another type of medication. His health care provider will look at what other medications he is taking, what other health conditions he has, and any allergies he might have before making a decision on drugs.

Here are some of the drug options that health care providers are using to help arthritis sufferers find relief:

• *Biological response modifiers.* These new drugs, such as Enbrel and Remicade, are used for the treatment of

g a
a so
has
the

hritis to reduce inflammation in the

i-inflammatory drugs (NSAIDs). These
rugs including aspirin and ibuprofen
educe pain and inflammation and may
a short-term and long-term relief in
eoarthritis and rheumatoid arthritis.

Iay

clude Celebrex, one of the so-called
rs that block an enzyme known to
atory response.

ease,
these
s, no
have
ed at
killers
hon-
n and
e, that

ese are hormones that are very ef-
arthritis but cause many side effects.
n be taken by mouth or given by in-
e is the corticosteroid most often
to reduce the inflammation of
is. In both rheumatoid arthritis and
doctor also may inject a corticos-
ected joint to stop pain. Because
may cause damage to the cartilage,
e only once or twice a year.

s, such
e man
ress of
a man
, espe-
e pain
s value
nto his

uronic acid products like Hyalgan
a naturally occurring body sub-
tes the knee joint and permits
ment without pain. A blood-
d the Prosorba Column is used in
lities for filtering out harmful an-
h severe rheumatoid arthritis.

urgery is the only real option. The
n an operation to remove the
y), realign the joint (osteotomy),
place the damaged joint with an
lasty). Many men say that al-

though they were reluctant to have surgery, havi
total joint replacement has provided them wit'
much relief that it literally changed their lives. I
gotten them back up and active again, often fo
first time in years.

What Alternative Lifestyle Therapies N
Relieve Arthritis Pain?

Many people seek other ways of treating their di
such as special diets or supplements. Although
methods may not be harmful in and of themselv
research to date shows that they help. Some peopl
tried acupuncture, in which thin needles are inser
specific points in the body to release natural pain
(endorphins). Others have tried glucosamine and
droitin sulfate, two natural substances found i
around cartilage cells, for osteoarthritis of the kne
can be found over the counter in pharmacies.

Some alternative or complementary approache
as acupuncture or magnetic therapy, may help tl
in your life cope with or reduce some of the s
living with a chronic illness. It is important that
tell his doctor if he is using alternative therapie
cially over-the-counter medications to manage t
and symptoms. If the doctor feels the approach h
and won't harm him, it can be incorporated i
treatment plan.

Exercise and Arthritis

Excess pounds put extra stress on weight-bearing joints such as the knees or hips. Studies have shown that some individuals who lost an average of eleven pounds substantially reduced the development of osteoarthritis in their knees. In addition, if osteoarthritis has already affected one knee, weight reduction will reduce the chance of it occurring in the other knee.

Building exercise into his routine can really help him manage his arthritis. It can not only help take the pounds off but also help to relieve some of the pain and stress on the joints, improve his muscle strength and flexibility, and improve his cardio endurance. A value-added feature of adding an exercise program is that he may lose weight, which means he is putting less stress on his hip, knee, and ankle joints, thereby making him more mobile and reducing the pain.

Sports and fitness trainer Nina Moore says that it is vital for a client to consult with his physician before starting an exercise program. Once he gets permission from his doctor, she says that she works with him to create a program of exercises and stretches that can improve his range of motion, and then introduce some low-impact aerobics. "Swimming and water aerobics are excellent for someone living with arthritis because they don't put stress on the joints."

She suggests that her clients add in strength building exercise by using weights. "I always tell them not to try to do too much at a time, and use small weights successfully before going to the next level." Nina says that taking on a routine that is too strenuous, too rapidly can do more harm than good for a man living with arthritis.

ALZHEIMER'S DISEASE

Jeannie and Willie Collier looked forward to retirement. They've had a long and wonderful life together. "He was my high school sweetheart," she says of the man she's been married to for more than fifty years. They raised six children together.

The Colliers had sacrificed and saved and worked to be financially secure in their future. They hoped to travel a little and visit their adult children and grandchildren and just take it easy. Then Jeannie started to notice small changes in Willie. "He'd forget things. He'd get quiet around the children because he knew he was forgetting, but didn't want anybody to notice. And he stopped reading. Willie had always been an avid reader of books on black history almost all his adult life. "You'd almost never see him without a book, or ready for a debate on something or other," Jeannie says.

"We'd been thinking about retiring, and putting it off," Jeannie says. "Then one day Willie came in from work and said that he was so confused. He told me he was having a hard time remembering how to do tasks at work." She says it was clear that he had been having some minor problems here and there, but when he came to her in that way, she knew that it was time to do something.

It was at that moment that the decision she'd been struggling with became crystal clear. "I had to retire to take care of my husband," she says. The diagnosis of Alzheimer's disease changed their world.

The progression of the disease has had its ups and downs. "In the beginning there were good days and bad days, but now it seems like the days are a little rougher," she says. Willie now has difficulty with everyday tasks, and much of Jeannie's day is devoted to attending to his needs. He doesn't remember people on a regular basis anymore, just Jeannie.

They are committed to living in the house that they built together for as long as they can. One of their sons lives with them and provides daily support like cooking meals and house repairs so that Jeannie can concentrate on Willie's care. Another son lives down the street and checks in regularly. Willie doesn't remember exactly who they are most days. "He calls my son who lives here 'the man who lives in the basement,'" Jeannie says with a chuckle, because she says she's had to develop a real sense of humor lately. "You just learn to go with it," she says.

What Is Alzheimer's Disease?

Back in the day, before we had a name to attach to it, everybody knew some elderly person who was "not quite there." Warchal Faison, MD, from the University of Mississippi, an expert on Alzheimer's disease, says the medical community is just now starting to recognize and acknowledge that it is something other than just being senile. "We'd say that Grandpa was a little off. He'd wander off. He'd hide money or food and forget where he had hid it. Sometimes he would remember people and places. Sometimes he wouldn't. Before we had a name to call it, we just wrote Grandpa off as being a little crazy," Dr. Faison says. But she adds that Alzheimer's is not a mental illness.

Black Americans are disproportionately affected by the disease. The Alzheimer's Association suggests that the prevalence may be anywhere from 14 percent to a staggering 100 percent higher than that among white Americans. While Alzheimer's is not a disease that happens just because a person gets old, age does play a role. Under ordinary circumstances, sixty-five seems to be a magic number in Alzheimer's disease among black Americans. The chance of developing Alzheimer's doubles every five years after the age of sixty-five.

Alzheimer's is the most common form of dementia, a group of diseases that slowly destroy brain cells. Alzheimer's disease interferes with the way the brain's neurotransmitters send messages to each other. Eventually the disease causes nerve cell death and tissue loss, literally shrinking the brain. There is no cure.

Patrick Griffith, MD, is head of neurology at the Meharry Medical School, and is a leading specialist in Alzheimer's in people of color. He says that many black men are being diagnosed later, meaning that they struggle for years before they receive an accurate diagnosis and effective treatments that could forestall the effects of the disease. The progression of the disease can take anywhere between three and twenty years or longer.

A study released in 2006 by the Alzheimer's Foundation of America says that nearly 60 percent of family members or caregivers reported a delay in getting a diagnosis, due to shame, stigma, and living in denial experienced either by themselves or the person living with the disease.

In its early stages diagnosing Alzheimer's disease can be difficult. The changes that a person experiences, such as lost keys or forgetting where he parked the car, can be very subtle. But as the disease progresses, most families start looking for answers with their family practice physician or internist who will probably refer your family member to a doctor with specialized experience in diagnosing and managing the care of a person living with Alzheimer's and other kinds of dementia. In a specialized medical center, such as the one Dr. Griffith works in at Meharry that has professionals experienced in the diagnosis and treatment of the disease, diagnosis is accurate 90 percent of the time.

Medical researchers, like Dr. Griffith and Dr. Faison, don't have a concrete answer as to why black men and black women are affected by Alzheimer's at such high rates. It's difficult to pinpoint or even obtain accurate numbers of people living with the disease because blacks are not well represented in the past and current research. The research does suggest that there are ties between Alzheimer's and cardiovascular diseases such as plaque buildup and high blood pressure. They do know that blacks have a higher incidence of vascular disease and a higher incidence of vascular dementia. Black Americans are the largest minority group who are over sixty-five. And 65 percent of black recipients of Medicare B have hypertension, which is linked to the disease.

Treatment

As we have said, there is no cure for Alzheimer's but there are drugs that are being used for patients with mild to moderate forms of the disease. Dr Griffith says that prescription medications such as Namenda and Aricept can slow the progression of the disease for a period of time for a patient in the earlier stages, but currently nothing will stop it. "These drugs can make it possible for a person living with the disease to stay at home longer." But he adds that it is not a long-term solution.

He says that one drug, BiDil, does hold some promise specifically for black patients. "More research needs to be done, but it suggests that we need to explore how medications affect different races and ethnicities," Dr. Griffith says. But he adds that it has been difficult to make much progress because black patients are less willing to become involved in clinical trials.

How Long Can a Person with Alzheimer's Stay at Home?

The big question with any loved one living with Alzheimer's disease is how long can he live at home and be supported by caregivers? Each situation is an individual one. Some people do not have a person who can commit him- or herself to being an around-the-clock caregiver like Jeannie.

Others like Mildred Edmonds start out making a strong commitment to provide in-home care for their parent as long as they can, but eventually have to make a tough decision to place their loved one in a nursing facility that may be better equipped to handle the growing needs of an advanced Alzheimer's patient.

"Someone told me that being a caregiver seemed to be killing me and they were right. We had my father with me for eight years, and I just couldn't do it anymore," Mildred says. "It was a hard decision, and I felt a lot of guilt, but I had no choice," she says. Her father passed away after two years in a nursing care facility.

Can He Prevent Alzheimer's?

There is no vaccine or magic bullet out there to prevent or cure Alzheimer's. Experts like Dr. Faison suggest that the best thing a man can do for his health is to control his blood pressure and keep his cholesterol levels in check, since they think there is a link between these two conditions and Alzheimer's. It's not lost on us that yet again, the prevention tips for almost every disease that affects people of color are true for the prevention of Alzheimer's, too. Go back and review the tips we give you for controlling these two conditions in other sections.

In addition, experts feel that it is important to do all you can do to keep the mind and memory active. They recommend activities that require brainpower, like working puzzles, engaging in hobbies and crafts, and reading. They also recommend that as men age, it is important to continue to have stimulating social contact.

According to researchers at Duke University's

African American Community Outreach Program, there does seem to be a familial link to the disease. Their data suggest that nearly half of all first-generation relatives of black Alzheimer's patients are at some risk for getting the disease themselves. The Alzheimer's Association says that blacks who have a first-generation relative who has or had the disease are at over 43 percent risk of developing dementia themselves. And in the largest study of black Americans with Alzheimer's the data showed that there was an 18.4 percent risk of developing the disease if you were the spouse of a patient, because you were sharing the same environmental factors that may have triggered the disease.

What Are the Warning Signs of Alzheimer's Disease?

Sheila Jack, who is the associate director of diversity outreach for the Alzheimer's Association, says she and her family know firsthand about the ravages of the disease. She lost her father to Alzheimer's. "It was in the 1980s when we didn't think about Alzheimer's. We just thought he was acting crazy." She says he was also young when he started exhibiting symptoms. Sheila recounts an episode where they were attending a family reunion. "He just wandered off. We found him later in a diner having pie and drinking coffee," she says. He died in his sixties. "We didn't really know that he had Alzheimer's until after his death, after they did an autopsy." Even though experts in the field of geriatric medicine can do a good job of diagnosing Alzheimer's, the only definitive way to know for sure is an autopsy that looks at the brain of the person.

Mildred Edmonds says that her father, a widower, was always meticulous about his appearance. "A natty dresser," she says. He was active as a deacon in his church for over twenty years. He paid his bills on time. "Then one day it seems that all that changed. The bills stacked up. He started missing church. And he wasn't well put together anymore," Mildred says.

Dr. Faison says that these symptoms are common and calls the progression of the disease the "longest good-bye." She says that an Alizheimer's patient loses bits and pieces of himself a little at a time. She says it is not uncommon for a man to forget the names of his spouse or his children as he slips further into the disease. A person suffering from Alzheimer's may do so for three to twenty years after diagnosis. Because diagnosis is often made in later stages, it becomes difficult to give a "typical" answer of how long a person will live with the disease.

Alzheimer's slowly steals a person's thinking and memory capacity. It never seems to happen at once, but a little bit at a time. Dr. Faison says that in the earliest stages there are really few differences between a person with Alzheimer's and the rest of us who are struggling to remember what we did with our car keys. Later, a person becomes a little more forgetful. He may have a hard time coming up with the right word for something.

As the disease progresses, a person can't perform simple tasks that he has done in the past. Slowly the person loses more and more of his memory and ability to do things for himself, including feeding and bathing.

The warning signs of Alzheimer's by themselves can be the same symptoms many of us experience as we age. But when you add them up, it may be time to seek help from a doctor or a geriatric nurse who has experience in assessing the disease. The average time between the first symptoms and warning signs and a diagnosis is two years or more.

Here are some of the warning signs of Alzheimer's disease:

- Memory loss
- Misplacing things regularly
- Problems with use of common language
- Confusion about time and place
- Impaired judgment
- Difficulty in performing routine tasks such as dressing himself
- Loss of interest in things that he was once passionate about, such as hobbies, his appearance, social activities

What Can We Do to Slow Down or Stop the Progression of the Disease?

As we've discussed, the bad news is that once a person starts the slippery slope of living with Alzheimer's there is no cure, and there is nothing at this point that will stop it in its tracks. The medications Aricept and Namenda can slow the disease's progression. Each works differently, and there is "no one size fits all" solution. Some drugs have been known to cause nightmares and headaches in some people. Dr. Faison says it can be trial and error to find out what works with any one individual. These medications tend to work best in the earlier stages of the disease.

"Most black men who suffer from Alzheimer's are diagnosed in the later stages when the medications are least effective," Dr. Faison says, but adds that there are real advantages to getting a diagnosis earlier. "Having a diagnosis in the earliest stages gives families time to get a plan. It also gives the affected person, the man in your life, whether it is your husband, or your father, or uncle, a chance to be a part of the planning process," she says.

Because many families live in denial about what is going on, they don't use the precious time in the early stages of the disease to prepare for the time when the person can no longer make decisions about his financial affairs, or how he would like to be cared for. Then suddenly (or what feels like suddenly), family members scramble to create caregiving support systems for that person. That's why Dr. Faison says that getting a diagnosis and making plans early on is important.

Taking action earlier also gives the person who is living with Alzheimer's and his family a chance to learn more about the disease and its progression. There are almost always major decisions that need to be made for the future of the person living with Alzheimer's. Who will be his caregiver? What financial decisions need to be made? Who will the person live with? What kinds of modifications does the house or apartment need?

What You Really Need to Know . . .

Black women play a huge role in the support of a loved one living with the disease. Three out of four Alzheimer's caregivers are women. And we are more likely to keep our loved ones at home to care for them. If you are a caregiver, family member, or part of a support system for a father, husband, or friend living with Alzheimer's, you really have to change your thinking about life with that person. "Things will never be the same," Jeannie says. But she deals with it gracefully day by day.

There is a lot of stress and frustration for caregivers of a man living with Alzheimer's. Jeannie says it is important to remember that the person is not faking, acting out, or deliberately trying to get on your nerves. She adds, "It takes a lot of patience—every day."

Again, education is key for caregivers, says Dr. Faison. What seemed logical yesterday is not necessarily logical today. Jeannie and her six adult children have had to learn that Willie is not going to change, because he can't. It is the other family members who have to adapt and change when one family member develops Alzheimer's.

Ask any woman who has been a caregiver or support system for a love one with Alzheimer's and she will tell you that it is the most painful thing to watch and live through. There is nothing, even if you have read everything you can read, and talked to everyone you can talk to, that will really prepare you in an up-front and personal way for this disease. It's one thing to read about what other families have gone through, but when your father doesn't remember who you are, it takes on a whole new meaning. Education is key for the man living with Alzheimer's and those entrusted with his care. Utilize the excellent resources that are now available.

CHAPTER 14

End-of-Life Care

Richard Payne, MD, started his medical career wanting to save lives, but moved into a branch of medicine that few were talking about or addressing—what happens when we reach the end of our lives. Dr. Payne is one of the leading experts in the world on pain and palliative care and end-of-life issues, and is the director of the Duke Institute on Care at the End of Life at Duke University. He says that "the biggest risk factor for death is being born, or in other words, death is a natural part of life."

Dr. Payne tells a story that hits close to his home. He talks about a call he received from a family member about another relative who had many health issues that required his attention and care. "He had diabetes, high blood pressure, high cholesterol. He was obese, and he didn't exercise or follow any of the recommendations his health care provider had set out if the relative wanted to improve his health and his ability to live as long as possible," he says. When the inevitable call came that his relative had a stroke and was in bad shape, he was saddened, but not surprised. He was also not surprised to find out that there was no advanced planning done on his relative's behalf.

Dr. Payne says these are hard conversations to have and challenging subjects to think about. If we feel uncomfortable talking about issues of health and staying well, we all know how difficult it is to talk about preparing to die. Throughout this book we have been talking about many of the challenges of getting a black man we love to take better care of himself. So we wrestled with the idea of adding information about end-of-life care issues to a book about getting and staying well, and came to the conclusion that it was essential.

Black men have fears that keep them from being self-directed in their health care. Their fear of being diagnosed with cancer prevents them from scheduling yearly screening. Fears keeps them from following through on lifestyle changes that will prolong their lives like eating healthier, taking their meds to control their high blood pressure and diabetes, and giving up cigarettes. But their fears also keep them from having an end-of-life plan. Yes, it is hard to face your mortality.

Dr. Payne suggests that the very best time for planning and making decisions on who determines your care when you can't speak for yourself is way before it is needed. He suggests that these decisions and the paperwork that goes with them are done in advance of any health crisis. In fact, he and other experts recommend getting the forms and filling them out when you are feeling fine. Nobody ever really knows when he will no longer have the power to speak for himself. If you've ever been involved in these family discussions when a loved one has gotten a terminal diagnosis, or is in a coma, you know how emotional and painful these situations can be. At a time when families are dealing with their fears of losing the person, they are suddenly being asked to make decisions on how the person will spend the last months, weeks, or days of his life.

A few years ago everything that could go wrong did in Florida, in the much publicized Terri Schiavo case. What was normally handled as a private family matter became a headline grabber and fodder for the courts that lasted for years. Dr. Payne says that out of the drama that had the nation stunned, the one thing the Schiavo case did for the rest of us is to show how important it is to make your medical-care wishes known. Legal and medical experts say that at the height of attention in the media to that case, there was a dramatic increase in individuals and couples having discussions with their family members and requesting living will and advanced directive forms.

GET A PLAN

Every person needs a living will and an advanced directive long before it is necessary. Having these documents in place before they are needed is not like bringing bad luck your way, it just means that you are prepared for whatever life throws you and that you have taken the time to make decisions on the way you will manage your health. When you talk about creating a way to be in control of your life and your health care, just know that advanced planning is as important as taking your medicines or selecting the right doctor. It gives you your say.

Forms are available on the Internet that can guide you through the process, but it is probably worth it to consult with your family attorney, who will be aware of what is specifically required in your state and community, and will know exactly where your paperwork needs to be sent.

Every adult has the right to make a decision on getting or refusing medical care. The man in your life has the right to say, "No, I do not want to receive this type of treatment," or "Yes, I want treatment." As long as he is alert and what is considered competent, it is his legal right to make those decisions for himself. Experts define competent as having the ability to understand your condition and the results the decision you make may have.

If faced with tough decisions, a man's medical team should be giving him the information he needs on his condition and the next steps in treatment, as well as the best medical advice possible. Legally, as long as he is competent, he is the only person who can make these important decisions.

But here is one of the things that can often cause problems. As long as the person is considered competent, he (or she) has the right to refuse treatment. He gets to say "no" to treatment, even if it may keep him alive longer or if his doctor or family members want him to continue with treatment.

Where it really gets difficult is when he becomes too sick to make his own decisions. Without an advanced directive or living will, decisions get made for him, whether they are the decisions he would have want to be made or not. The bottom line is without direction from him, no one will know what he would have decided on his own behalf. Having those instructions in place through a document called an advance directive (AD) gives you a voice in making key decisions.

WHAT IS AN ADVANCE DIRECTIVE?

Advance directives are documents that an adult person signs when he is still able to give direction to his health care providers and his family about what treatment he wants or does not want under certain conditions. It is a document that speaks for him, at a time that he can't speak for himself.

A durable power of attorney for health care ("durable power") is a type of advanced directive document that names a specific person to act as his "patient advocate" to act and speak on his behalf to carry out his medical wishes. This person's job as the patient's advocate is to make sure that the person's medical wishes are carried out. One of the challenges for anyone who is willing to step up and act as a patient advocate is to remember to advocate the patient's wishes, not the advocate's personal value system.

A living will is different. It allows a person to put his wishes for his care in writing, but it does not name a specific person to advocate on his behalf. While most

ecide
o this
ld be
g not
rning
ter.
 situ-
.e sit-
tions.
tional
resus-
inally

ity, or
ent to
e de-
:ment
levas-
ble to
    with

:Y

nding
.e any
e his
on his
ortant
ishes,
erson

ot have either, people who work in
at families should consider having
you have the wishes of the patient
and a designated person, often a
will fight for his right to have those
oring a do not resuscitate (DNR)

un Advance Directive?

ng, why turn something so private
nething that sounds so legal? We all
s have been born and died in this
s of years without an AD or any
And if a black man has a wife or
adult children whom he trusts to
ions on his life, then why would he
mal as a document to tell people

families can be unpredictable. For
be torn between what they knew
rother wanted and what they per-
st and most moral thing to do. We
one who has strong feelings about
want to receive or refuse in certain
ve an advanced care planning in
ible. If your father knows that he
ept alive for a long period of time
ling tubes, then he needs to make
e known.
on that should happen between

couples or in families early on. He should be free to
who will make these decisions for him, if he can't c
for himself. It could be his spouse, but it co
someone else for a number of reasons, includir
wanting to put the heavy burden of such things as tv
off life support on a spouse who might feel guilty l

This idea of directing care in these health crisi
ations is frightening. It is not the most comfortak
uation for anybody. But they are important convers:
Together you should talk about his feelings on add
surgeries, drugs, feeding tubes and ventilators, or
citation. What would he want if he became tern
ill, or was unconscious and not likely to wake up?

What if he were suffering from dementia, seni
Alzheimer's and could not be considered compet
make these decisions? The best time to make the
cisions and decisions on what kind of medical trea
he would want if he ever suffered a stroke, or a
tating medical condition that made him totally una
care for himself, is before he and you are facec
them.

DURABLE POWER OF ATTORN

A durable power of attorney is a legally bi
document that allows the man in your life to nar
person who is eighteen years old or older to
patient advocate and make health care decisions
behalf. When picking a patient advocate it is imp
to have someone that he trusts to carry out his v
and not act on his or her own value system. The

that he selects should actually be willing to serve in that capacity. It sounds simple, but not everyone is willing to have that kind of life-and-death pressure on them.

A durable power can be used to accept or refuse any treatment. If he wants his patient advocate to be able to refuse any treatment and let him pass away without extraordinary interventions, he must say so directly in the durable power document. As his patient advocate, you can only make those decisions for him if and when he cannot make those decisions for himself.

Nobody absolutely has to have a durable power of attorney document. An individual can write down his wishes and share them with his doctor and family members. But, the patient advocate has no legal standing to make decisions, in the case of conflict, without this document.

HAVING THE CONVERSATION

As Dr. Payne says, "The best time to start putting plans in place for a living will and or an advanced directive is way before it has to be put into action." Needless to say, it makes sense to start having those conversations early and often.

You may think you know what the man in your life wants, but you could be wrong. It isn't unusual to be engaged in a casual conversation, only to find out that he has a totally different idea of what he wants to have happen than you do, or than you think he does. These are not always easy conversations to have. Nobody likes to talk about illness or health crises or death.

Dr. Payne says that many of the best opportunities to begin these conversations occur at church or in a community meeting. "Churches are realizing that this is a valuable part of their health ministry. And it is a natural place to start." Of course, much of the real work of making these decisions happens at home.

Many men choose to have this very personal discussion with their significant others. But in many cases the discussions include other family members, as well. While the discussions of advanced care are private and individual, having them with the family members who may have to carry out the wishes, or may get revved up to fight a decision, may prevent confusion and hard feelings among adult children and their siblings and other family members later.

Sharon Latson, the national director of Outreach Among Communities of Color at Vitas Hospice, has been encouraging families to acquire a better understanding of the advanced planning options available to them. There is a wonderful document called Five Wishes that is being used to guide many families of color through the process. It is offered through Aging with Dignity at www.agingwithdignity.org and is free. It gives you all the steps you and your family need to make these important decisions.

Have several copies made and keep them ready to go. In order for your paperwork to be legally binding, it must be witnessed and signed by a party who is not a family member, or the health care provider. In addition, keep a copy with the important papers and make sure that others have copies that they can get to quickly in case of an emergency.

Advance care planning is not etched in stone. The man in your life can change his mind at any time about the decisions he has laid out. Experts like Dr. Payne and Sharon Latson agree that it is a good idea to review your decisions and make changes, if you see fit, once a year. There are lots of reasons that he may want to make changes. His views on the decisions he made the year before may have changed. His health situation may be different. The person he designated as his patient advocate may no longer be able or willing to serve in this capacity. A review will give him a chance to plan accordingly.

LET THE CHURCH SAY AMEN . . .

A few years back, when some of the black churches were first discovering the need for advanced planning and end-of-life care, Deacon Rosalyn Priester, of Trinity United Church of Christ in Chicago, Illinois, worked with Sharon to obtain 1,000 of the Five Wishes documents, customize them with quotes from Trinity staff and community residents, and add the phrase "Embracing Amani" on the front of the cover. *Embracing Amani* means "the ultimate healing and peace of atonement with God."

Deacon Priester announced the Advanced Directive Day Workshop in the church bulletin, on the Web site, via the phone, mailings, and in the church newsletter. About fifty residents from the community and members of the church attended the workshop. They viewed the training video and filled out the document. Community residents continued to engage in conversations on end-of-life care well into the evening.

The doors are now open to these conversations in our community, but we have to work to keep them open.

HOSPICE CARE/COMPASSIONATE CARE

As we discussed, we really do see this as a health book that highlights ways to keep our men stronger and living longer, and so we debated writing about end-of-life care and hospice. Of course, we would rather you and the men in your life focus on being as well as you can be. But at some point you may be faced with end-of-life care needs for someone you love. We want you to have a bit of this information too.

What Is Hospice Care?

Hospice care is end-of-life care that is supported by a holistic medical team including a medical director, nursing staff, spiritual support in many cases, and a host of volunteers. Just like almost every other aspect of health care there are big gaps in access and use of hospice and end-of-life care for black individuals and families. One of those reasons is that the idea of facing death and dying is a very hard thing to do. It feels like letting go.

Best-selling historical romance author Beverly Jenkins suddenly became the primary caregiver for her husband, Mark, after he was diagnosed with what ended up being terminal lung cancer. Beverly and Mark had been together since 1971. "I did it all, including hosting mini-wakes for Mark and his friends as they came over to say their good-byes," she says. "My priest told me that I had raised the bar on caring for a loved one at the end of his life. But I told him that I know Mark would have done nothing less for me."

Mark and Beverly made the decision together to utilize hospice services as a way to keep him comfortable and at home until the end, which is what they both wanted. "He'd always hated hospitals," she says.

Beverly says that hospice was an invaluable resource because the team also helped him manage his pain and managed all the physical issues that go along with a person dying from cancer, like need for oxygen. "Hospice was wonderful."

If you have been caring for a loved one for a period of time, but are not now able to keep him comfortable, and free from pain (which is one of the main things we want at the end of life), it feels like something broke. Suddenly what you did yesterday for the person you love is not working today.

Hospice often feels like failure for family members. It can feel like throwing in the towel, because it means that you have given up hope—or so it seems. But Dr. Gwendolyn London, a minister and expert in compassionate care at the end of life, says that "bringing in hospice support is not a sign of failure, it is in fact a gift. It can help free you up from the day-to-day stresses of pain management and other technical aspects of your loved one's care. It gives you a chance to spend real quality time together to love each other, talk honestly to each other, and to say good-bye."

Latson says that one of the reasons that black families have a hard time accepting this kind of outside help is that it is historically a very private time. People might go to the hospital or hospice facility to have outside care, but the idea of bringing strangers into the home to help out is hard to accept.

It is taking a while for families to get used to and to embrace hospice, but Dr. Payne says it is happening. "The more families who have a positive experience that honors their culture and values, the more the word of mouth will spread on the benefits of using either in-home or facilities-based care."

Finding good, compassionate hospice care, thank goodness, has become easier in the past ten years. The best place to start is with your loved one's doctor or nursing staff. They have lots of experience most times with what is available in your area. And think about using hospice services sooner rather than later. Unfortunately, many families make the decision to use hospice in the very late stages of a person's life. It is not uncommon for a person to die shortly (hours or days) after being moved to a hospice facility or after introducing hospice care into the home.

Epilogue

In *The Black Woman's Guide to Black Men's Health* we've shared stories, given you the facts and figures and some very specific tips that you can use to help the men in your lives be healthier and live longer. And even though we all know that getting a black man to be proactive about his health and preventing serious illness is a huge challenge, the inspiring stories we've shared have shown you that is has been done and is being done every day. With just very small efforts, black women are getting their men to the doctor; and they are helping them make changes that, hopefully, they will be able to keep for a lifetime. As many men will tell you, black women are saving lives because they won't take no for an answer.

The book is full of recommendations—some big and some small. You may not be able to do all of them in a day; in fact, you shouldn't even try. Take it in baby steps. Do what you can do today to make some of the changes, and then a little more tomorrow. And if you are at a loss as to where to start, the key is not where you begin, but that you *do* begin. Perhaps the best place to start is with a conversation, as we describe in chapter 1.

The key is to remember that you are helping him, you are not managing him, you are not taking over, you are not running his business. You are helping him, because you love him and you want him around for a very long time.

The point is that every single black woman can have a major impact on the health of the men in her life. And if his wife or girlfriend, mother, sister, grandmother, and friends all tag team him, he is definitely a brother bound for change.

In fact, we each have the strength, creativity, and power to touch the lives of many black men who need our nurturing and care—whether they realize it yet or not. We like to call it the true power of one . . . one woman, one church, one family of strong black women, and one community with one goal—to get our black men back on track with their health. Every single black woman has a role to play—many roles to play. We want to share some ways that collectively black women can make a difference beyond the men in our lives, but for all black men, today and in future generations. We all know the power of one person, but can only dream of the possibilities for our people if we join forces. Following are some things you can do to make an impact on a larger scale.

WHAT ONE CHURCH GROUP
CAN DO . . .

- Start a health ministry if your church does not have one. Make sure that it is an active part of the church.
- Create faith-based health initiatives, host educational health programs and regular screenings for high blood pressure, diabetes, and prostate cancer.
- Encourage the physicians, nurses, psychologists, and social workers in your congregations to get involved in providing health care to the uninsured and under-insured.
- Bring in speakers from the medical profession to talk to the congregation on days other than Sunday. Host conversations around living wills, advanced directives, long-term care, and end-of-life care.
- Create a health information resource library. Get members to donate books about chronic disease, med-ications, etc. Start a health navigators program. Find the people in the church who are willing to be the "go-to" people for information on programs, health care providers, community offerings, etc.
- Talk about HIV and AIDS prevention, detection, and support. There are people in almost every church in this country who are either living with HIV/AIDS or are at risk (both men and women).

WHAT ONE SORORITY, SOCIAL OR COMMUNITY SERVICE ORGANIZATION, OR GROUP OF GIRLFRIENDS CAN DO . . .

- Conduct health fairs.
- Host a Black Men's Health event for women in the community. Think about partnering with other groups to ensure that you get a crowd.
- Support programs and initiatives that target key issues for men and women of color.
- Enlist the help of the black beauty salons, barbershops, car washes, and hangout spots in spreading the word. If black men won't go to the information, bring the information to them.
- Use some of your scholarship funds to help support young men and women of color who are working toward a career in the medical and health professions.

WHAT ONE COMMUNITY CAN DO . . .

Sandra Gadson, MD, is the president of the National Medical Association and a nephrologist. In both her roles she sees the costs our community is paying for health care disparities. "Access is a big issue," Dr. Gadson says. "There is a shortage of community health centers; hospitals are closing and reducing services." She sees that these closings coupled with not having the funds or insurance to pay for care will put our communities at even more risk.

Dr. Gadson says we have to take ownership of what's happening in our communities around access to care. According to Dr. Gadson we all need to be prepared to speak up and advocate for access to care.

Some of the things we can do in our communities to protect services and increase access for our men and ourselves are:

- Talk to our public officials about the need for more health care options in our communities.
- Vote for candidates who are as concerned about the issues that affect health, such as employment, housing, education, health care benefits, the availability of fresh, nutritious foods. Support candidates who are against environmental hazards, such as toxic waste that causes cancer, in communities of color.
- Support no-smoke zones in restaurants and public places, and funding for smoking cessation outreach and education that is culturally appropriate for men of color.
- Insist upon physical education programs in every school, and the reduction of soft drinks in school vending machines. Both contribute to childhood obesity and early onset diabetes in school-age children of color. Support school-based health center programs for our youth.
- Help to create a safe and healthy environment in public housing in your community. Look at successful models from other communities.
- Do not accept campaigns that are geared toward black men, but are not culturally effective. Be prepared to call them on it.

• Push for racial and ethnic diversity training in your health and medical institutions. Insist that your health service organizations and policymakers have some people of color on staff who will help shape programs and services that will affect us.

WHAT OUR BLACK FEMALE LEGISLATORS CAN DO . . .

• Continue to fight against health care disparities through legislation and funding.
• Continue to work for improved access to health care for black men and women regardless of ability to pay.
• Begin to address the health issues of black men who are incarcerated and will one day re-enter our communities.
• Vote for increased funding for outreach and awareness campaigns, testing sites, school-based health centers, etc.
• Hold more legislative briefings on the issues of health, gender, and race.

It seems that we have put a lot of pressure on ourselves to make big changes in the health and well-being of men. By now you have got to be asking what black men should be doing for themselves. Some might say that the best thing they can do to be healthier is to listen to us. But the best thing they can really do is be as diligent about their health as they are about sports and hanging out with the fellas. They can understand that taking steps to take care of themselves is a matter of life and death. We know that black women have an awful lot of work to do to make this happen, but individually and collectively we will make a difference.

So we urge you to be proactive. Not just in your home, in your family, in your relationships. We want you to help us create a movement of black women working to affect the lives of black men for now and the future. We can create such a buzz and flex such big muscle power on this one, even if it is with our gentle persuasiveness. And together, let's promise to do something— lots of something. Our men need us.

We'd love to know what you are doing as you go about helping to make a difference. Share your stories with us at www.andreacollier.com.

Important Health Resources

Here are some helpful resources that can help you navigate care for the men in your life.

CHAPTER 1: *Getting Started*

Men's Health Network
www.menshealthnetwork.org
202-543-6461

Sickle Cell Disease Association of America
www.scdaa.org
410-528-1555

CHAPTER 2: *Financing Health Care*

Community Voices
www.communityvoices.org

AARP
www.aarp.org
1-800-OUR-AARP

Medicaid
www.cms.gov
1-877-267-2323

Medicare
www.medicare.gov
1-800-MEDICARE (1-800-633-4227)

Health Assistance Partnership
www.healthassistancepartnership.org
202-737-6340

Georgetown University Health Policy Institute
Offers a state by state guide of health insurance programs addressing how to get health insurance coverage, and how to keep it.
www.healthinsuranceinfo.net

Health Guides USA
www.healthguideusa.org

CHAPTER 3: *Finding the Right Doctor*

The American Medical Association
www.ama-assn.org
1-800-621-8335

The National Medical Association
www.nmanet.net
202-347-1895

CHAPTER 4: *Prescription Drugs*

Together Rx Access
www.togetherrxaccess.com
1-800-444-4106

Partnership for Prescription Assistance
www.pparx.org
1-888-4PPA-NOW

RxAssist
www.rxassist.org

RxHope
www.rxhope.com

The AARP Guide to Pills
MaryAnne Hochadel (Sterling, 2006)

CHAPTER 5: *For the Record*

United States Surgeon General's Family Health History Initiative
www.hhs.gov/familyhistory

Centers for Disease Control
www.cdc.gov

CHAPTER 6: *Obesity*

Centers for Disease Control and Prevention's Obesity Information
www.cdc.gov/nccdph/dnpa/obesity

American Dietetic Association
www.eatright.org
1-800-877-1600

American Obesity Association
www.obesity.org
202-776-7711

Weight Watchers
www.weightwatchers.com

Donna Richardson Joyner, *Sweating in the Spirit*
www.donnarichardson.com

Healthy Cooking Magazines

Cooking Light, www.cookinglight.com

Essence, www.essence.com

Ebony, www.ebony.com

Healthy Cookbooks

Patti LaBelle's Lite Cuisine
Patti LaBelle and Laura Randolph Lancaster
(Gotham, 2004)

Healthy Food, Healthy Soul: African American Cooking
Kenda E. Tibbs (Kenda Tibbs, 1999)

The New Ebony Cookbook
Charlotte Lyons (Johnson Publishing, 1999)

The Diabetes and Heart Healthy Cookbook
The American Diabetes Association and the American
Heart Association (American Diabetes Association
2004)

Black Family Dinner Quilt Cookbook
Dorothy Height (Fireside, 1994)

*Hallelujah! The Welcome Table: A Lifetime of Memories
and Recipes*
Maya Angelou (Random House, 2004)

CHAPTER 7: *Cardiovascular Diseases*

The American Heart Association
www.americanheart.org
1-800-242-8721

The American Stroke Association
www.americanstroke.org
1-800-242-8721

National Stroke Association
www.stroke.org
1-800-STROKES

CHAPTER 8: *Diabetes*

www.diabetes.org
1-800-DIABETES

National Institute of Diabetes, Digestive and Kidney Diseases
www.niddk.nih.gov

CHAPTER 9: *Cancer*

American Cancer Society
www.cancer.org
1-800-ACS-2345

National Cancer Institute
www.cancer.gov
1-800-4-CANCER

NCI 5 a Day Program
www.5aday.gov

Centers for Disease Control Screen for Life Campaign
www.cdc.gov/cancer/screenforlife

Colon Cancer Network
www.colorectal-cancer.net
301-879-1500

Colon Cancer Alliance
www.ccalliance.org
1-877-422-2030

The Stennis Family Foundation
www.stennisfamilyfoundation.org
1-866-965-2220

American Lung Association
www.lungusa.org
1-800-LUNGUSA

Prostate Cancer Foundation
www.prostatecancerfoundation.org
1-800-757-CURE

National Prostate Cancer Coalition
www.fightprostatecancer.org
1-800-245-9455

US TOO Prostate Cancer Information
www.ustoo.com
1-800-80-US-TOO

That Black Men Might Live
Rev. Charles Williams and Vernon Williams
(Hilton Publishing, 2003)

The American Academy of Dermatology
www.aad.org
1-866-503-SKIN

Doctors Approach
www.doctorsapproach.com

CHAPTER 10: *Mental Health*

The American Psychiatric Association
www.psych.org
703-907-7300

The American Psychology Association
www.apa.org
1-800-374-2721

National Association of Black Social Workers
www.nabsw.org
202-589-1850

National Center for Primary Care
www.msm.edu/ncpc.htm
404-756-5740

Carter Center Mental Health Program
www.cartercenter.org
404-420-5100

Depression and Bipolar Support Alliance
www.dbsalliance.org
1-800-826-3632

National Institute for Mental Health
www.nimh.nih.gov
1-866-615-6464

National Alliance for the Mentally Ill
www.nami.org
1-800-950-6264

Standing in the Shadows: Black Men and Depression
John Head (Broadway, 2004)

*Lay My Burden Down: Unraveling Suicide and the
Mental Health Crisis Among African Americans*
Alvin Poussaint, MD, and Amy Alexander
(Beacon Press, 2001)

CHAPTER 11: *Oral Health*

American Dental Association
www.ada.org
312-440-2500

CHAPTER 12: *Let's Talk About Sex*

The Black AIDS Institute
www.blackaids.org
213-353-3610

Balm in Gilead
www.balmingilead.org
1-888-225-6243

National Black Leadership Commission on AIDS
www.nblca.org
1-800-992-6531

Centers for Disease Control
www.cdc.gov
1-800-CDC-INFO

National Institutes of Health
www.aidsinfo.nih.gov

National HIV Testing Resources
www.HIVtest.org
1-800-HIV-0440

Books and Magazines

*Real Health,*www.realhealth.com

Poz, www.poz.com

Sexuality and the Black Church: A Womanist Perspective
Kelly Brown Douglas (Orbis Books, 1999)

CHAPTER 13: *Aging*

Arthritis Foundation
P.O. Box 7669
Atlanta, Georgia 30357-0669
www.arthritis.org
1-800-568-4045

The National Institutes of Health's National Institute of Arthritis and Musculoskeletal and Skin Diseases
www.niams.nih.gov

The Alzheimer's Resource Room
www.aoa.gov

The Alzheimer's Foundation of America
www.alzfdn.org
1-866-AFA-8484

The Alzheimer's Association
225 N. Michigan
Chicago, Illinois 60601
www.alz.org
1-800-272-3900

The National Institute on Aging, Alzheimer's Disease Education and Referral Center
http://www.nia.nih.gov/alzheimers
1-800-438-4380

National Family Caregivers
www.nfcacares.org
1-800-896-3650

Family Caregivers Alliance
www.caregiver.org
1-800-445-8106

CHAPTER 14: *End-of-Life Care*

Five Wishes, Aging with Dignity
www.agingwithdignity.org
1-888-5-WISHES

Duke Institute on Care at the End of Life
www.iceol.duke.edu
919-660-3553

Hospice Foundation of America
www.hospicefoundation.org
1-800-854-3402

National Hospice and Palliative Care Organization
www.nhpco.org
1-800-658-8898

Vitas Hospice
www.vitas.com
1-800-93-VITAS

Still with Me ... A Daughter's Journey of Love and Loss
Andrea King Collier (Simon & Schuster, 2003)

Index

About the Authors

Andrea King Collier is a freelance journalist, who specializes in health and health care. Her work has appeared in *O* (the Oprah Magazine) *Essence, More, Ladies' Home Journal, Better Homes and Gardens, Women's Day, Real Health,* and others. Collier's first book, *Still with Me: A Daughter's Journey of Love and Loss,* is a memoir about her journey as a caregiver. Collier lives in Lansing, Michigan.

• • •

Willarda V. Edwards, MD, MBA, is the president and chief operating officer of Sickle Cell Disease Association of America, Inc. (SCDAA). She is formerly the national director of the NAACP Health Advocacy Division. Dr. Edwards holds a degree in medicine from the University of Maryland Medical School in Baltimore,

Maryland, and a master's in business administration from Loyola College in Baltimore. She is also a practicing internist in Baltimore, Maryland. Dr. Edwards has served on the board of trustees of the National Medical Association for over twelve years and has served as chairman of the board.